Promoting Healthy Behavior:

How Much Freedom? Whose Responsibility?

Hastings Center Studies in Ethics

A SERIES EDITED BY

Mark J. Hanson and Daniel Callahan

This series of books, published by The Hastings Center and Georgetown University Press, examines ethical issues in medicine and the life sciences. Established in 1969, The Hastings Center, located in Garrison, New York, is an independent, nonprofit, and nonpartisan research organization. The work of the Center is mainly carried out through research projects, the publication of the *Hastings Center Report* and *IRB: A Review of Human Subjects Research,* and numerous workshops, conferences, lectures, and consultations. *The Hastings Center Studies in Ethics* series brings the ongoing research of The Hastings Center to a wider audience.

Promoting Healthy Behavior:

How Much Freedom?
Whose Responsibility?

EDITED BY
Daniel Callahan

GEORGETOWN UNIVERSITY PRESS / WASHINGTON, D.C.

Georgetown University Press, Washington, D.C. 20007
© 2000 by Georgetown University Press. All rights reserved.
Printed in the United States of America
10 9 8 7 6 5 4 3 2 1   2000
THIS VOLUME IS PRINTED ON ACID-FREE OFFSET BOOK PAPER

Library of Congress Cataloging-in-Publication Data
Promoting healthy behavior : how much freedom? whose responsibility? /
    edited by Daniel Callahan.
        p.   cm. — (Hastings Center studies in ethics)
    ISBN 0-87840-762-6 (cloth : alk. paper)
    1. Health promotion—Social aspects. 2. Health promotion—Moral
and ethical aspects.   I. Callahan, Daniel, 1930–   .   II. Series.
RA427.8.P766   2000
613—dc21   99-38856
                                                    CIP

CONTENTS

Preface

This book is the result of a two-year research project on the ethical and social dilemmas of health promotion and disease prevention. The project was carried out jointly by The Hastings Center and the Stanford University Center for Biomedical Ethics. It was supported by grants from The California Wellness Foundation and the Walter & Elise Haas Fund of San Francisco. We are particularly grateful to Barbara Koenig, executive director of the Stanford Center, and to her colleagues for their help in the organization of the project and for serving as hosts of our meetings in California. Meredith Minkler was enormously helpful in identifying just the right people for the project. We also want to thank Mark Hanson of The Hastings Center for his work in preparing this book for publication. The authors of the papers in the volume were all participants in the project. They were an interesting, lively, and informative group, and we all profited from our time together.

Daniel Callahan

Introduction

Health promotion and disease prevention seem, on the surface, to present few social and ethical problems. No one speaks against them, the media and legislators feel kindly about them, health maintenance organizations (HMOs) have embraced them, and most of the available health care statistics seem powerfully to support them. Yet for all their rhetorical momentum, in practice they fall far short of the high hopes invested in them. Obesity is up, exercise is down, teenagers continue to be drawn to smoking, and sexually transmitted disease goes on in its not-so-merry way. What's wrong? What's being missed?

The research project that led to these papers was designed to explore those questions and the puzzles behind them. There is no shortage of innovative and experimental projects to change poor health behavior; indeed, such efforts have spawned an active and committed enterprise. There are, however, or seem to be, fewer explorations of the ethical and social problems that may be putting subtle and hidden obstacles in the way, than the enterprise—and its mixed record of success—requires.

Our premise is this: It is a mistake to see health promotion and disease prevention simply as instances of educational and technical challenges. There are such challenges but, as a movement, health promotion and disease prevention raise some profound questions about the role of the state or employers in trying to change health-related behavior, the actual health and economic benefits of even trying, and the freedom and responsibility of those of us who, as citizens, will be the target of such efforts.

We selected for examination some key questions about these matters, commissioned a number of papers, and spent a great deal of time going over and arguing about early drafts of those papers. Meredith Minkler's paper opens this collection by focusing on a question that must be pursued if there is to be any serious progress in health promotion and disease prevention: Just how free are we, as individuals, to shape our behavior and to live healthy lives? Are we all equally free (or equally unfree) or does our social and economic context make a difference?

Beverly Ovrebo carries those concerns into the legal arena, examining the pressures that new and widespread diseases place on traditional public health practices (often draconian in the past) but now situated in a society more sensitive to civil liberties and uncertain how to balance severe health risks against potentially severe threats to liberty in trying to control them. It is an old story but with some strikingly new developments.

But what if health promotion and disease prevention programs succeed? Would they actually save money, as is commonly said? Helen Halpin Schauffler takes up that question in a direct and unsparing way. She argues not only that it is a myth to think that money will be saved, but also that the health promotion movement is harmed by efforts to make this kind of case, one that too often entails unwarranted hyperbole and some outright deception. E. Haavi Morreim addresses a related issue, that of the moral legitimacy of using economic and other incentives to bring about behavior change, and usually (as with HMOs) for the specific purpose of holding down the costs of health care.

Ann Robertson and Ronald Labonte, our Canadian contributors, brought to the discussion the fruits of a long and intense debate on public health in their country, a debate in many ways far richer than anything yet to take place in the United States. What they bring to the foreground is the necessity of setting health promotion and disease prevention efforts within the broader context of the ethos and politics of a nation. By arguing for a communitarian perspective, they show that efforts to improve the health of the public must be deeply rooted in a view of human nature and human societies. Barbara Koenig and Alan Stockdale show most effectively how the powerful scientific drive for greater genetic knowledge, and the exploitation of the uses to which it can be put, will almost certainly force a confrontation among a number of our settled social values. In particular, they argue that an increase of tension can be expected between the idea that people should be held responsible for their genetically related health behavior and the more wide-ranging implications of scientific development that bring out the importance of environment in shaping behavioral and genetic outcomes.

In my essay I explore a question that intrigued me greatly as our project progressed. Could it be that our society is fundamentally ambivalent about health promotion and disease prevention, and that the source of that ambivalence is the powerful libertarian strain that has historically run through our society. We want good health but we also want to be free of government meddling with our health. We like the idea of programs in health promotion but we are prepared to turn against them when they seem to pose threats to our personal choice of lifestyles. How might this tension be better dealt with? The final essay by Barbara Koenig, Meredith Minkler, and me represents the sum of what we learned from the project and where we believe health promotion and disease prevention programs need to go in the future. We argue that these programs are likely to be less than wholly successful unless they can be complemented by a fuller examination of their place in our national values and institutions.

MEREDITH MINKLER

Personal Responsibility for Health: Contexts and Controversies

When lifelong smoker Jean Connor died of lung cancer in 1995 at age forty-nine, her family brought a wrongful death suit against cigarette manufacturer R.J. Reynolds, arguing that Connor had been "lured into smoking" as a teenager by glamorous tobacco advertisements and was heavily addicted before cigarette warning labels made their appearance. The Florida jury, half of whose members currently smoked and one of whom was a former smoker, handed down a verdict in support of the tobacco company, whose lawyer had argued that "cigarette smoking is very much a matter of choice."

The personal responsibility verdict in this mid-1997 case was curiously timed, coming in the midst of a flurry of antitobacco sentiment and legislation and mounting public support for unprecedented crackdowns on an industry accused of deliberately marketing to children, increasing the nicotine content of cigarettes, and in other ways causing undue harm to the public's health.[1] Yet even as antitobacco-industry organizing reached landmark proportions in the United States, the dominant American ideology with respect to smoking—and any number of other "lifestyle factors" and health-related behaviors—remained heavily focused on personal rather than social responsibility for health.

Following a brief discussion of the contested meaning of "personal responsibility for health," this chapter will explore the current emphasis on personal responsibility, giving particular attention to the reemergence of interest in this concept of the late 1970s and its shaping of the dominant perspective on health promotion in the United States today. The case for a heavy emphasis on personal responsibility for health will be presented and contrasted with arguments that such an emphasis may "blame the victim," further stigmatize devalued groups (e.g., the elderly and disabled), oversimplify complex human behaviors, and ignore the mounting epidemiological evidence that individual behavior change can have only a limited impact on the distribution of disease in society. A case will then be made for a balanced approach stressing individual responsibility for health within a context of broader social change that enables increased "response-ability" on the individual level. The chapter will close by presenting the Canadian approach to health promotion developed in the mid-1980s and refined during the past decade as an example of a balanced approach that may constitute both good efficacious practice and "good ethics."

The Contested Meaning of "Personal Responsibility for Health"

As Daniel Wikler has argued, the seemingly simple premise that "individuals are responsible for their health" means very different things to different people.[2] The self-help or holistic health advocate who calls for wresting control of one's health from the traditional medical establishment is likely to hold a very different interpretation from that of the individual for whom personal control over health is fundamentally a moral question of right and wrong. To underscore and clarify these diverse perspectives, Wikler turns to Dworkin's typology of the several alternative meanings of responsibility in the debate over health promotion and personal responsibility for health.[3] The latter schema differentiates between *role responsibility* (one's body belongs to one's self), *causal responsibility* (one's health status is in large part determined by personal behavioral choices), and *responsibility based on liability* for costs and other "undesirable" consequences of one's illness.

Whereas "role responsibility" in this schema may imply nothing more than one's "role" as a biological organism, "causal responsibility" implicates the individual's choices and actions with regard to diet and exercise, for example, in helping to determine his or her health status. In the words of the Rockefeller Foundation's late president John Knowles, the "primary critical choice" facing the individual is thus whether "to change his personal bad habits or quit complaining. He can either remain the problem or become the solution to it."[4] Finally "responsibility based on liability" would suggest that the unhelmeted cyclist who sustains a head injury, or the smoker who develops lung cancer, bears responsibility for the medical care costs and other undesirable consequences of his or her "foolish behaviors."

As Wikler goes on to point out, depending on which interpretation of personal responsibility for health is adopted, one may invoke ethical or even judicial notions of paternalism, general utility, communitarianism, or fairness and compensation to inform policy choices regarding health and health promotion and disease prevention.

Each of these underlying conceptual orientations will be discussed in greater detail by others in this volume in relation to such contested health promotion policy issues as the use of economic and other incentives to modify health behavior, and the interface between health promotion and civil liberties. The salient point for this chapter, however, is that even among strong advocates of personal responsibility for health, profound albeit often unspoken disagreements may exist in the foundational assumptions concerning the meaning of responsibility in relation to individual health and health-related behaviors.

"Personal Responsibility for Health" in Recent Historical Perspective

Notions of personal responsibility for health have surfaced and resurfaced throughout human history. The effects of lifestyle on health were emphasized in ancient Greece and Rome, and the notion that individuals had at least some control over their health continued, to varying degrees, through the Middle Ages and the Renaissance.[5]

In the United States, as in other nations, several shifts in the assignment of responsibility for health have been put forward, with an emphasis on personal control and self-sufficiency emerging in the early 1800s and again toward the end of the nineteenth century. Despite such shifts, however, a dominant cultural preference for notions of personal responsibility has been noted throughout our history, which is consonant with the Jeffersonian democracy's emphasis on voluntarism, decentralization, and only limited obligation to the common good.[6]

The current dominant view of health promotion in the United States emerged in the 1970s in response to a growing disillusionment with the limits of medicine, pressures to contain health care costs, and a social and political climate emphasizing self-help and individual control over health.[7] It is a vision that sees individual behavior in large part as responsible for the health problems we face as a society. In the words of J.K. Iglehart, editor of *Health Affairs,* this vision suggests that "most illnesses and premature death are caused by human habits of living *that people choose for themselves*" (emphasis added).[8]

Ironically, this traditional approach to health promotion has tended to be disease oriented rather than health oriented. As Wallack and Montgomery have pointed out, it defines health primarily as the absence of disease, and considers disease as being associated largely with known and controllable risk factors such as cigarette smoking, poor diet, and heavy drinking.[9] The individual is seen as the appropriate focus for intervention to control risk factors, with those interventions typically consisting of providing knowledge and skills for changing unhealthy behaviors.

This vision of health promotion was given institutional expression in Canada with the publication of the Lalonde Report in 1974,[10] and in the United States in the Surgeon General's report, *Healthy People,* published in 1979.[11] Both of these documents, it should be noted, discussed the role of broader environmental factors in influencing health and did not limit themselves to a discussion of individual lifestyle or personal behavior issues. The Surgeon General's report, for example, argued persuasively that "we are killing ourselves," not only by "our own careless habits," but also by polluting the environment and permitting harmful social conditions to exist.[12] Despite their efforts to address some of these broader issues, however, the major contributions of both the Lalonde and the surgeon general's reports lay in calling attention to the often substantial role individuals can play in modifying their personal behaviors and in other ways improving their health status.[13]

In the United States, the surgeon general's report was followed by the development of clearly articulated and measurable "Objectives for the Nation."[14] The listing of activities for achieving each objective was extremely thorough and included strategies on the levels of institutional change, legislation and policy, and not merely in the realm of personal behavior change.

In reality, however, implementing this broad vision of health promotion, particularly in an era of fiscal conservatism, proved difficult indeed. Moreover, as Green has noted, the sharp distinction drawn in U.S. policy between *health promotion* (focused mainly on behavior and life-style issues) and *health protection* (concerned more with the physical environment) led to a narrower interpretation of health promotion in the United States than in many European nations, which argued that both physical and social environmental factors lay within the purview of health promotion.[15] In Green's words: "We Americans allowed our health promotion terrain to be restricted to lifestyle determinants of health, but we also allowed lifestyle to be interpreted too narrowly as pertaining primarily if not exclusively to the behavior of those whose health is in question."

As a consequence, most of the programs that grew out of the renewed push for health promotion and disease prevention in the United

States beginning in the late 1970s tended to focus primarily on the level of personal behavior change. The programmatic emphasis on individual *responsibility* for health, in short, frequently was not accompanied by attention to individual and community *response-ability,* or the capacity of individuals and communities to build on their strengths and respond to their personal needs and the challenges posed by the environment.[16] Following an examination of the case for and against a personal responsibility focus in health promotion, we will return to the notion of a balanced approach that stresses both individual responsibility and broader society action enhancing "response-ability."

The Case for Personal Responsibility for Health

The past three and a half decades have seen the amassing of an impressive body of evidence supporting the importance of individual responsibility for health.[17] Indeed, Daniel Callahan has argued that "nothing is more evident in the statistics of public health than the role played by individual health behavior in contributing to accidents, illness and disease."[18] In a now-classic series of studies, for example, Lester Breslow and his associates revealed that men who followed seven personal health habits—eating breakfast, drinking only in moderation, not smoking, and so on—had lower morbidity and mortality rates than those who followed six; those who followed six of the habits had better health and mortality outcomes than those who followed five, and so forth.[19] Similarly, Kayman and others demonstrated that individuals who develop their own diet and exercise plans are more successful at achieving and maintaining weight loss than those who play a more passive role.[20] Finally, when Michael McGinnis and William Foege calculated the leading causes of death for Americans under seventy-five, not by disease such as cancer, coronary heart disease, and stroke, but rather by putative or "actual" cause, tobacco, diet, and exercise—all factors directly related to individual behavior—were found to constitute the greatest causes of premature death.[21] The two most rapidly increasing causes of mortality—sexual behavior and illicit drug use—were also among those with strong behavioral components.

The case for a strong emphasis on personal responsibility for health is frequently built on the fact that there is much room for improvement in the health habits of Americans. The United States has record rates of obesity and eating disorders, and fully 35 percent of Americans were overweight in the mid-1990s.[22] More than 60 percent of adults are not physically active on a regular basis and 25 percent lead sedentary lives.[23]

While smoking rates dropped substantially from 40 percent in the mid-1960s to about 22 percent by the mid-1990s,[24] tobacco still accounts for well over 400,000 deaths per year, leading the Centers for Disease Control and Prevention to dub smoking "the most devastating cause of disease and premature death this country has ever seen."[25]

Finally, recent evidence suggests that the prevalence of some unhealthy behaviors has significantly increased over the last few years. Among eighth, tenth, and twelfth graders, for example, the proportion of youths who smoke daily increased by almost 50 percent between 1991 and 1996, with 20 percent of twelfth graders now smoking on a daily basis.[26] The proportion of adults who are overweight increased by 14 percent from 1980 to 1994,[27] and the proportion of high school students participating in daily physical education classes fell from 42 percent in 1991 to just 25 percent in 1995.[28]

Coupled with these and other indicators of the need for change is some impressive evidence that individual behavior change can achieve improved health outcomes. Each year, millions of smokers successfully quit the habit (albeit usually after three to four attempts), and most who do quit do so on their own.[29] For those individuals who need help in making lifestyle modifications, increasingly sophisticated behavior change techniques and interventions have sometimes resulted in high success rates. The Stanford Coronary Risk Intervention Program (SCRIP), for example, which combined comprehensive lifestyle modification in terms of diet, exercise, and smoking with counseling and medication, reported a 40 percent lowering in cholesterol consumption, a 23 percent reduction in low-density lipoproteins (LDL), a 20 percent increase in exercise, and other significant changes over a four-year period. Although both groups in this randomized clinical trial experienced some worsening of their heart disease and three died in each group, the SCRIP participants demonstrated 47 percent less narrowing of their arteries and had only slightly more than half the number of hospitalizations of the controls.[30] Numerous smaller-scale interventions stressing lifestyle modification also have demonstrated success.[31]

Research on successful lifestyle modification programs for the elderly has also been important in demonstrating that despite a troubling health profile (70 percent of Americans over sixty-five are sedentary, 16 percent smoke, and 20 percent are overweight), many older Americans both choose to participate in such programs and have low recidivism rates following smoking cessation and other lifestyle changes.[32] The Los Angeles-based Medicare Screening and Health Promotion trial (MSHPT) thus boasted participation rates of over 70 percent ($N = 1,911$) with no significant differences at baseline in the health habits and behaviors of participants and nonparticipants. Although this trial was limited to a largely white, middle-class community, the finding of comparability in health behaviors between those elders who took part and those who did not suggests that health promotion and disease prevention efforts may effectively reach those for whom personal behavior changes could make a significant difference in terms of risk factor reduction.[33]

The above arguments are frequently cited as part of the scientific base for approaches to health promotion that stress personal responsibility. Yet another important part of this case is firmly grounded in ethics, since this perspective acknowledges human agency or individual will and choice in deciding on a course of action. In Callahan's words, "Most of the health habits of most of us are under our control. . . . At best we can argue mitigating circumstances, diminished response and mild victimization, but only a small minority can claim they lack responsibility altogether."[34] The human agency argument highlights the role of intentional or purposive action in health achievements.[35] Proponents of the human agency argument, for example, point to dramatic declines in cigarette smoking and consumption of saturated fats from the 1960s through the 1980s, with a corresponding decline by about one-third in deaths from coronary heart disease and stroke over that same period.[36] Although it is impossible to determine the extent to which these dramatic declines in stroke and heart disease mortality can be attributable to personal behavior changes in diet and smoking, the death rates from both diseases began to fall well in advance of the widespread use of pharmacological agents.[37] Examining the evidence in this regard, Jack Farquhar has suggested that personal decisions to change health behaviors must indeed be credited with some of the declines observed—a perspective that again highlights the human agency argument.[38]

As Neubauer and Pratt have noted, notions of "the freedom to think and to act, to exert control over situations, to gain respect from others—all on one's own terms," are particularly important to Americans and make the human agency component of the dominant approach to health promotion a compelling one.[39] Intimately related to the notion of human agency is the idea that individuals have a fundamental right, based on the principle of autonomy, to choose health-related behaviors. Yet with this right, so the argument goes, comes a responsibility to make "wise" choices. A major assumption of the human agency argument, with particular relevance in relation to the responsibility side of this equation, involves the notion that individuals can make choices in relative isolation from the broader social environment of which they are a part. In Larry Churchill's words, such thinking is embedded in "a moral heritage in which answers to the question 'what is good?' and 'what is right?' are lodged definitively in a powerful image of the individual as the only meaningful level of moral analysis."[40] Yet as Robert Bellah et al.,[41] Sandel,[42] and others make clear, the moral actions of individuals (and, I would argue, their health-related actions) can only be understood in a broader social context. It is to this and other critiques of the dominant notion of "personal responsibility for health" that we now turn.

The Case "Against" Personal Responsibility for Health

Though few would argue that individuals bear no responsibility for health-related decisions and actions, several consistent criticisms have been leveled at what many see as the dangers of an overemphasis on individual responsibility for health. Foremost among these criticisms is the argument that an overriding emphasis on personal responsibility "blames the victim" by ignoring the social context in which individual decision making and health-related action takes place.[43] In the words of Rob Crawford, the victim-blaming ideology "both ignores what is known about human behavior and minimizes the importance of evidence about the environmental assault on health. It instructs people to be individually responsible at a time when they are becoming less capable as individuals of controlling their health environment."[44]

Holding the individual responsible for health choices is particularly problematic in the case of the poor, since poverty itself is now widely accepted as among the most significant risk factors for illness and premature death.[45] Mary Haan and her colleagues, for example, demonstrated in their study in Alameda County, California, that residence in a poverty neighborhood resulted in a 40 percent excess mortality rate.[46] Significant differences in mortality remained even when smoking, diet, exercise, and other traditional risk factors were controlled for.

Increasing scholarly effort has been devoted to elucidating those mediating factors that may explain the relationship between personal responsibility and socioeconomic status (SES). Central to much of this theorizing and research is the notion of control as a "transcendent concept" that can help explain health outcomes and health behaviors at both individual and broader population levels.[47] Epidemiologist S. Leonard Syme has suggested, for example, that people at progressively lower socioeconomic levels have correspondingly less opportunity to control the circumstances and events that have an impact on their lives.[48] Conversely, for individuals at higher SES levels, factors like higher income and greater discretion, and latitude and control over decision making at work may contribute to a more generalized sense of "control over destiny," which in turn may translate into enhanced health behaviors and health outcomes. Other theorists, while often operationalizing terms differently, have come to similar conclusions. Indeed, as Syme has noted, "loss of control has been defined in terms of constraints on coping ability, diminished authority over decisions, threats to status and self-esteem, lessened opportunity to learn new skills, and inappropriateness of coping."[49] The concept has been variously used further in reference to perceived control and actual control, and to control as a state of being and as a condition under which things are "in control." Despite (or perhaps because of) the wide range of definitions and measurement tools employed, the notion of control is increasingly seen as having value in helping to explain the link between unhealthy behaviors and poor health and SES.[50]

Separate yet often intimately related to SES are other aspects of the social context in which individual health behavior takes place that must also be considered in any discussion of personal and social responsibility for health. We have long known, for example, that SES "is transformed by racism,"[51] with race differences in quality of education, income, returns on education, and costs for goods and services such as housing, food, and automobile insurance.[52] Further, as Robison has pointed out, even after controlling for work experience and education, employed African Americans are exposed to more occupational hazards and carcinogens than are whites.[53]

We are only beginning to appreciate, however, the more subtle impacts of racism as a risk factor for heart disease, depression, and other illnesses.[54] And only with the advent of a movement for environmental justice have we begun to appreciate the health consequences of such inequities as the fact that people of color have incinerators placed in their neighborhoods at a rate 89 percent above the national average.[55] The implications of such findings are troubling, and they suggest the need for far more serious attention to the racial/ethnic and related aspects of the social environment in which health-related behavior takes place.

Finally, the cultural environment in which individuals are expected to take personal responsibility for their health must also be thoughtfully considered. The average school-aged child, for example, watches 10,000 television commercials per year, and in a single recent year, W.K. Kellogg spent $32 million advertising a single product—Sugar Frosted Flakes.[56] During that same year, the amount spent by the U.S. government on nutrition education for school children was just $50,000 per state.[57] On an even larger scale, as Robison points out,[58] when our culture continues to say to us, "why walk when you can ride?" and when it admonishes us to get every new labor-saving device and not even leave our chair to change a television channel, or our computer to send a fax; is it any wonder that the notion of building in forty minutes three or four times a week for exercise goes against the grain? When these broader environmental contexts and realities are taken into account, the limitations of an approach to health promotion based on personal responsibility for health are cast in stark relief.

Another important dimension of the victim-blaming potential of an overemphasis on personal responsibility for health involves the fact that by equating "being ill" with "being guilty," we may inadvertently stigmatize the disabled, the elderly, people who are overweight, and other already devalued groups in our society.[59] The renewed emphasis on individual responsibility for health thus has been accompanied by the reemergence of a Victorian era notion that healthy old age is a just reward for a life of self-control and "right living."[60] In David Levin's words, "good health has become a new ritual of patriotism, a marketplace for the public display of secular faith in the power of the will."[61] In such a vision, where is the place for the eighty-five-year-old man with a disabling respiratory ailment or the obese and severely arthritic elderly woman in a wheelchair?

Caroline Wang similarly has demonstrated that health promotion approaches to injury prevention that stress personal responsibility and carry the implicit or explicit message, "Don't let this happen to you!" often inadvertently stigmatize people with disabilities, suggesting that they are "inherently flawed" and undesirable.[62] She poignantly quotes a paraplegic who, on viewing a series of ads depicting people in wheelchairs with scare-provoking captions said, "It feels like I should be preventing myself!" In cases like these, an overemphasis on individual responsibility for the state of one's body or health may inadvertently contribute to messages that reinforce ageism, handicappism, and other prejudices.

Another widely held criticism of the heavy emphasis placed on individual responsibility for health involves the argument that such a perspective lets government "off the hook" by assigning blame for premature morbidity and mortality and the like to the individual. Frequently underlying this criticism is the fact that conservative governments have used the rhetoric of personal responsibility for health to justify cutbacks in needed health and social programs.[63] The Personal Responsibility and Work Opportunity Reconciliation Act of 1996,[64] which repealed America's sixty-year-old commitment to welfare entitlement for the poor and, by some estimates, may throw more than a million additional children into poverty,[65] is a classic example. The political use—and misuse—of the language of individual responsibility to support programs and policies like this one may be devastating in their human costs and consequences.[66]

Critics of an overemphasis on personal responsibility for health also frequently invoke an epidemiological argument, pointing out that encouraging individual behavior change can have only limited impact on the distribution of disease in communities.[67] Two factors contribute to this reality. First, getting people to maintain a behavioral change over time, like cutting back their intake of high-fat, high-calorie foods, or sustaining an exercise regimen, is difficult. Half of all individuals who begin an exercise regimen quit within six months, for example, and "weight cycling" among individuals who repeatedly fall off their diets is an extremely common problem that can have both adverse psychological consequences in terms of feelings of failure and physiological ones.[68] Studies have shown marked increases in coronary heart disease as well as elevated all-cause mortality among weight cyclers, even when such other factors as smoking are controlled for.[69] Such facts underscore the complexity of the behaviors that must be altered if people are to achieve and maintain weight loss, nonsmoking status, and other desired health outcomes. As one researcher put it, personal responsibility approaches that compare giving up smoking and other unhealthy behaviors to "just saying no" to a scone at a tea party trivialize the difficulty of such sustained actions.[70]

In addition to the difficulty of behavior change maintenance, epidemiologists point out that given the sheer prevalence of diseases such as lung cancer, heart disease, and stroke, solutions focused on individual responsibility for change are unlikely to have much effect. Each year, for example, 4.5 million people in the United States are newly diagnosed with coronary heart disease;[71] each day, six thousand teens smoke their first cigarette and another three thousand enter the ranks of "regular smokers"—those who smoke at least one cigarette daily.[72] Given such realities, a personal responsibility approach "does little to alter the distribution of disease in the population because new people develop disease even as sick people are cured and because new people enter the 'at risk' population as others leave it."[73]

Critics of the personal responsibility approach to health promotion also point to the limited effectiveness of many of the large, well-funded programs that have focused on individual behavior change. In the Multiple Risk Factor Intervention Trial (MRFIT), as Syme points out, "highly motivated men in the top 10 percent risk category for coronary heart disease were able to make only modest changes in their eating and smoking behavior in spite of intensive intervention over a six-year period."[74] Similarly, the widely touted COMMIT (Community Intervention Trial for Smoking Cessation) project, which represented the most ambitious and sophisticated antismoking program ever attempted, achieved only modest results.[75] It is important to note that many of the key architects of these ambitious efforts, which focused heavily on individual behavior change, are now among the most articulate spokespersons for the need for a broader environmental or societal responsibility focus. Stanford Heart Disease Project founder Jack Farquhar thus strongly advocates for increased excise taxes on cigarettes which, he argues, could reduce smoking rates far more effectively than individual change approaches.[76] Similarly, Syme, one of the world's foremost authorities on coronary heart disease and a lead researcher in the MRFIT program, now advocates approaches that stress community empowerment and increased social responsibility.[77]

Increasing evidence suggests that macro-level or environmental interventions, grounded in notions of social responsibility for health, can exert a powerful effect in changing behaviors on a broad scale. A 10 percent increase in the price of cigarettes, for example, has been shown to decrease teen smoking by 14 percent, and it is projected that a $2 per pack tax would decrease adolescent tobacco use by almost 46 percent.[78] Similarly, in their first few years of operation, reductions in the speed limit to fifty-five and mandatory seat belt laws cut automobile fatalities by more than all the preceding years of voluntary driver education programs combined.[79] Such facts and figures are compelling, and they bring us back to the epidemiological argument that only by focusing on broader environmental forces rather than on individual behavior change can we hope to have much impact on the distribution of disease in society.

Among the many criticisms that have been leveled at the ideology of personal responsibility for health, one of the least frequently discussed involves the observation that the personal responsibility argument is, in fact, applied in an extremely arbitrary fashion. As Faith Fitzgerald has pointed out,

> We excoriate the smoker but congratulate the skier. Yet both smoking and skiing may lead to injury, both may be costly, and are clearly risky. We have created a new medical specialty to take care of sports injuries, an acknowledgment of the hazardous sequelae. And though there are no doubt benefits to exercise and sports, the literature on the complications of some activities is such that were they drugs, they would probably have been banned by the Food and Drug Administration long ago.[80]

When certain lifestyles are branded socially unacceptable and others worthy of praise, even though both may lead to disease and dysfunction, an approach to health promotion that stresses "personal responsibility for health" must be carefully examined in terms of the ethical questions it raises.

A final and related dimension of the case against too strong an emphasis on personal responsibility for health involves the argument that through such an emphasis we risk establishing a "tyranny of health,"[81] in which, in Marshall Becker's words,[82] we substitute "personal health goals for more important, humane, societal goals." The dangers inherent in "healthism," which places health itself at the center of a new morality and elevates it to the level of a primary virtue, is discussed at length by Daniel Callahan elsewhere in this volume and will not be covered here. But the cautions that have been raised against health becoming "the paramount value of our society" should be seen as constituting still another important rationale for broadening the focus of our health-promotion approaches beyond those concerned with individual responsibility and lifestyle modification to acknowledge and attend to the larger environmental forces that must be addressed if healthier societies are to be attained.[83]

Balancing Individual and Social Responsibility for Health

As epidemiologist S. Leonard Syme once wrote:

> No one would argue that, as individuals, we are responsible for our health. In the final analysis, we are the only ones who can change our behavior. We are the only ones who lift fork to mouth, who inhale smoke, who plant feet on sidewalk. And we are the only ones who can *decide* to do these things. . . . [But] we don't live in a vacuum. Whether we like it

or not, our thoughts, ideas, wishes and behaviors are influenced and conditioned by the people around us, by the environments in which we find ourselves, and by the customs, traditions, fads and fashions to which we are continuously exposed. . . . Effective behavior change therefore requires that we do our best as individuals, but also that we work together with one another to create more healthful and supportive social environments.[84]

Working together means, I believe, balancing the notion of individual responsibility for health with a commitment to enhancing individual and community "response-ability." Toward the end of seeking a more balanced approach to health promotion—one that stresses personal responsibility for health within a context of broader social responsibility—it is useful to review the World Health Organization (WHO) vision of health promotion, and how that vision was crafted into a conceptual framework for health promotion policy and its implementation in Canada.

In the mid-1980s, WHO radically revised its notion of health promotion by defining it as "a process of enabling people to increase control over, and to improve their health." It went on to state that health promotion represents "a mediating strategy between people and their environments, synthesizing personal choice and social responsibility in health."[85] The principles set forth by WHO as underlying this alternative vision of health promotion included acting on the determinants or causes of health, eliciting high-level public participation, and using a variety of approaches that go well beyond lifestyle education and include legislation, organizational change, and community development.[86]

The Canadian approach to health promotion, which also was developed in the mid-1980s, provides an illustration of how such a broadened vision may constitute a useful framework for action. After a period of considerable preoccupation with healthy lifestyles and individual responsibility for health, the Canadian government undertook a massive restructuring of its approach to health promotion. Two important points stand out in the approach that was born of this restructuring. First, the number one challenge set forth for health promotion was reducing inequities between low- and high-income groups, and this was not framed in terms of individual responsibility but of broader societal responsibility.[87] Second, three levels of concern were set forth—health challenges, health-promotion mechanisms, and implementation strategies—and on each of these levels attention focused on the role of broad institutional or environmental change. Self-care, for example, was advocated within a framework that devoted considerable attention to the creation of healthy environments within which positive personal health behaviors could flourish. Canadian legislation on smoking, for example, is among the toughest in the world, with many provinces having developed "healthy public policies" on tobacco that have included changing their policies on marketing, crop substitution, and smoking in the workplace, at the same time that they urge individuals to quit the habit. Efforts to stop the tobacco company sponsorship of cultural and sporting events are also underway.[88]

In several Canadian provinces, a Premier's Council on Health has been established, through which government leaders in the different sectors provide advice on health promotion and work together to set goals to help address the social determinants of health.[89] Throughout Canada, hundreds of cities have designated themselves "healthy communities," stressing intersectoral planning, high-level community participation, and reciprocity between the individual and the broader society. And in the Northwest Territories, land claims and the development of First Nation's People's rights have been discussed as part of a broadly defined health agenda.[90] Hard outcome data that would indicate whether the new Canadian approach to health promotion will result in actual declines in morbidity and mortality are not yet available. Further, as Irving Rootman[91] and Lawrence Green[92] predicted, increased government perceptions of a need for cutbacks in social spending have led to some redesign of social programs in ways that are constricting the implementation of health promotion, in much the same way that cutbacks occurred in the United States under the Reagan and Bush administrations. Although the Canadian Public Health Association's recent "Action Statement for Health Promotion in Canada" reaffirmed the importance of continuing to use the Ottawa Charter as "the framework that defines health promotion in Canada," it went on to note that the current climate of increasing poverty, "global economic practices that imperil the environment," and cuts in the very health and social services that have defined Canadians "as a caring people" present a stark contrast to "the optimistic days when the Ottawa Charter was first written."[93] The Action Statement went on to reaffirm those visions and values deemed essential to health promotion, among them an "explicit value base" which includes the following precepts:

- Individuals are treated with dignity and their innate self-worth, intelligence and capacity of choice are respected.

- Individual liberties are respected, but priority is given to the common good when conflict arises.
- Participation is supported in policy decision making to identify what constitutes the common good.
- Priority is given to people whose living conditions, especially a lack of wealth and power, place them at greater risk.
- Social justice is pursued to prevent systemic discrimination and to reduce health inequities.
- Health of the present generation is not purchased at the expense of future generations.[94]

As noted earlier, even health-promotion efforts that are firmly grounded in a values base like this one may stumble as a result of continuing budget cuts, growing power differentials between rich and poor, and the structural distinctions that continue to exist between communities and health and social service professionals. At the same time, however, the Canadian framework for health promotion and the values and principles underlying it stand as an important example of a vision that offers a balanced concern for personal behavior change, within the context of broader social change. As the United States moves into the twenty-first century, the time is ripe for seeking such a balance in our nation's approaches to health promotion and disease prevention.

NOTES

1. Hubert H. Humphrey III, "Let's Take the Time to Get It Right," *Public Health Reports* 112 (1997): 378–85.

2. Daniel Wikler, "Who Should Be Blamed for Being Sick?" *Health Education Quarterly* 14, no. 1 (Spring 1987): 11–25.

3. Gerald Dworkin, "Voluntary Health Risks and Public Policy," *Hastings Center Report* 11, no. 5 (1981): 26–31.

4. John Knowles, ed., "The Responsibility of the Individual," in *Doing Better and Feeling Worse: Health in the United States* (New York: W. W. Norton 1977), p. 78.

5. Stanley J. Reiser, "Responsibility for Personal Health: A Historical Perspective," *Journal of Medicine and Philosophy* 10, no. 1 (1985): 7–17.

6. Reiser, "Responsibility for Personal Health"; Susan Noble Walker, "Health Promotion and Prevention of Disease and Disability among Older Adults: Who Is Responsible?" *Generations* (Spring 1994): 45–50.

7. H. M. Leichter, *Free to Be Foolish: Politics and Health Promotion in The United States and Great Britain* (Princeton, N.J.: Princeton University Press, 1991); Meredith Minkler, "Challenges for Health Promotion in the 1990s: Social Inequities, Empowerment, Negative Consequences, and the Common Good," *American Journal of Health Promotion* 8, no. 6 (1994): 403.

8. J. K. Iglehart, "From the Editor: Special Issue on Promoting Health," *Health Affairs* 9, no. 2 (1990): 4–5.

9. Lawrence Wallack and K. Montgomery, "Advertising for All by the Year 2000: Public Health Implication for Less Developed Countries," *Journal of Public Health Policy* 13, no. 2 (1992): 76–100.

10. M. Lalonde, *A New Perspective on the Health of Canadians* (Ottawa: Government of Canada, 1974).

11. U.S. Surgeon General, *Healthy People: The Surgeon General's Report on Health Promotion and Disease Prevention* (Washington, D.C.: Department of Health and Human Services, 1979).

12. U.S. Surgeon General, *Healthy People.*

13. Trevor Hancock, "Lalonde and Beyond: Looking Back at 'A New Perspective on the Health of Canadians,'" *Health Promotion* 1 (May 1986): 93–100; Milton Terris, "Newer Perspectives on the Health of Canadians: Beyond the Lalonde Report," *Journal of Public Health Policy* 5 (1984): 327–37; Deane Neubauer and Richard Pratt, "The Second Public Health Revolution: A Critical Appraisal," *Journal of Health Politics, Policy and Law* 6, no. 2 (Summer 1981): 205–29.

14. U.S. Surgeon General, *Health Promotion/Disease Prevention: Objectives for the Nation* (Washington, D.C.: Department of Health and Human Services, 1980).

15. Lawrence W. Green, personal communication from author, 17 May 1988.

16. Eli Zimmerman, personal communication from author, 16 October 1980.

17. Lalonde, *A New Perspective;* U.S. Surgeon General, *Healthy People;* S. Kayman, W. Bruvold, and J. Stern, "Maintenance and Relapse after Weight Loss in Women: Behavioral Aspects," *American Journal of Clinical Nutrition* 52 (1990): 800–807; Lisa F. Berkman and Lester Breslow, *Health and Ways of Living* (New York: Oxford University Press, 1983); J. Michael McGinnis and William H. Foege. "Actual Causes of Death in the United States," *JAMA* 270, no. 18 (1993): 2207–12; Center for Disease Control and Prevention, The President's Council on Physical Fitness and Sports, *Physical Activity and Health: A Report of the Surgeon General* (Washington, D.C.: U.S. Department of Health and Human Services, 1994), p. 10.

18. Daniel Callahan, "Preventing Disease, Creating Society," *American Journal of Preventive Medicine* 2, no. 4 (1986): 205–08.

19. Kayman, "Maintenance and Relapse."

20. Berkman and Breslow, "Health and Ways of Living."

21. McGinnis and Foege, "Actual Causes of Death."

22. Centers for Disease Control, "Update: Prevalence of Overweight among Children, Adolescents, and Adults: United States, 1988–1994," *Morbidity and Mortality Weekly Report* 6, no. 9 (1997): 199–202.

23. Centers for Disease Control and Prevention, *Physical Activity and Health.*

24. "State Specific Prevalence for Cigarette Smoking—U.S. 1995," *Morbidity and Mortality Weekly Report* 45, no. 44 (8 November 1995): 962.

25. U.S. Department of Health and Human Services, Office on Smoking and Health, *Smoking, Tobacco and Health: A Factbook* (Washington, D.C.: General Accounting Office, 1989).

26. Thomas E. Novotny, "Smoking among Black and White Youth: Differences That Matter," *Annals of Epidemiology* 6 (1996): 474–75.

27. "Update: Prevalence of Overweight," *Morbidity and Mortality Weekly Report.*

28. Centers for Disease Control and Prevention, *Physical Activity and Health.*

29. M. C. Fiore et al., "Methods Used to Quit Smoking in the United States: Do Cessation Programs Help?" *JAMA* 263, (1990): 2760–65.

30. William Haskell et al., "Beneficial Angiographic and Clinic Response to Multifactor Modification in the Stanford Coronary Risk Intervention Project (SCRIP)," *Circulation* 85, no. 4 (1991): II-140.

31. Kenneth Pelletier, "A Review and Analysis of the Health and Cost-Effective Outcome Studies of Comprehensive Health Promotion and Disease Prevention Programs at the Worksite: 1991–1993 Update," *American Journal of Health Promotion* 8, no. 1 (September/October 1993): 50–61; Centers for Disease Control and Prevention, *Physical Activity and Health;* Jonathan Robison et al., "Obesity, Weight Loss, and Health," *Journal of the American Dietetic Association* 93 (1993): 445–49.

32. E. Kligman, "Preventive Geriatrics: Basic Principles for Primary Care Physicians," *Geriatrics* 47, no. 7 (1992): 39–50.

33. S. O. Schweitzer et al., "Health Promotion and Disease Prevention for Older Adults: Opportunity for Change or Preaching to the Converted?" *American Journal of Preventive Medicine* 10, no. 4 (1994): 223–29.

34. Callahan, *False Hopes: Why America's Quest for Perfect Health Is a Recipe for Failure* (New York: Simon and Schuster, 1998), p. 191.

35. Knowles, *Doing Better and Feeling Worse;* Wikler, "Who Should Be Blamed?"

36. *1993 Heart and Stroke Facts Statistics* (Dallas, Tex.: American Heart Association, 1992).

37. John Farquhar, "Keynote Address: How Health Behavior Relates to Risk Factors," *Circulation* 88, no. 3 (1993): 1376–80.

38. Farquhar, "Keynote Address."

39. Neubauer and Pratt, "The Second Public Health Revolution," p. 217.

40. Larry Churchill, *Rationing Health Care in America: Perceptions and Principles of Justice* (Notre Dame, Ind.: University of Notre Dame Press, 1987).

41. Robert Bellah, *The Good Society* (New York: Alfred A. Knopf, 1991).

42. Michael J. Sandel, *Liberalism and the Limits of Justice* (Cambridge: Cambridge University Press, 1982).

43. Minkler, "Challenges," John Allegrante and Lawrence Green, "Sounding Board When Health Policy Becomes Victim Blaming," *NEJM* 305 (1981): 1528–29; Neubauer and Pratt, "The Second Public Health Revolution."

44. Rob Crawford, "You Are Dangerous to Your Health," *International Journal of Health Services* 4 (1977): 671.

45. S. Leonard Syme, "Rethinking Disease: Where Do We Go from Here?" *Annals of Epidemiology* 6 (1996): 463–68.

46. Mary Haan, George Kaplan, and Terry Camacho, "Poverty and Health: Prospective Evidence from the Alameda County Study," *American Journal of Epidemiology* 125 (1987): 989–98.

47. Syme, "Control and Health: An Epidemiological Perspective," in *Self-Directedness: Cause and Effects Throughout the Life Course,* ed. J. Rodin, C. Schooler, and K.W. Shaie (Hillsdale, N.J.: Erlbaum Associates, 1990), pp. 213–29.

48. Syme, "Community Participation, Empowerment, and Health: Development of a Wellness Guide for California" (lecture presented at the 1997 California Wellness Foundation/University of California Wellness Lecture Series, Berkeley, Calif., October 1997).

49. Syme, "Control and Health."

50. Syme, "Control and Health."

51. David R. Williams, Risa Lavizzo-Mourey, and Rueben C. Warren, "The Concept of Race and Health Status in America," *Public Health Reports* 109 (1994): 29.

52. Williams et al., "The Concept of Race," p. 29.

53. Jonathan Robison, "Racial Inequality and the Probability of Occupation-Related Injury or Illness," *Milbank Quarterly* 62 (1984): 567–90.

54. Williams et al., "The Concept of Race"; L. W. Sullivan, "Effects of Discrimination and Racism on Access to Health Care," *JAMA* 266 (1991): 2674; R. J. Blendon et al., "Access to Medical Care for Black and White Americans. A Matter of Continuing Concern," *JAMA* 261 (1989): 278–81; V. N. Salgado de Snyder, "Factors Associated with Acculturative Stress and Depressive Symptomatology among Married Mexican Immigrant Women," *Psychology of Women Quarterly* 11 (1987): 475–88; Nancy Krieger et al., "Racism, Sexism, and Social Class: Implications for Studies of Health, Disease, and Well-being," *American Journal of Preventive Medicine* 9 (1995): 82–122.

55. Pat Costner and Joe Thornton, *Playing with Fire: Hazardous Waste Incineration.* 2nd ed. (Washington, D.C.: Greenpeace USA, 1993).

56. Kelly Brownell and C. G. Fairborn, eds., *Eating Disorders and Obesity: A Comprehensive Handbook* (New York: Builford Press, 1995).

57. Brownell and Fairborn, eds., *Eating Disorders.*

58. Robison, "Changing Health Behaviors: We Know What to Do to Be Healthy: Why Don't We Do It?" (a paper presented at the Art and Sciences of Health Promotion Conference, Orlando, Fla., October 1995).

59. Marshall Becker, "The Tyranny of Health Promotion," *Public Health Reviews* 14 (1986): 15–23.

60. Thomas Cole, "The Specter of Old Age: History, Politics and Culture in an Aging America," *Tikkun* 3, no. 5 (1988): 14–18, 93–95; Jae Kennedy and Meredith Minkler, "Disability Theory and Public Policy: Implications for Critical Gerontology," in *Critical Gerontology: Perspectives from Political and Moral Economy,* ed. Meredith Minkler and Carroll Estes (Amityville, N.Y.: Baywood Publishing, 1999).

61. David Levin, *Pathologies of the Modern Self* (New York: University Press, 1987).

62. Caroline Wang, "Culture, Meaning and Disability: Injury Prevention Campaigns in the Production of Stigma," *Social Science and Medicine* 3, no. 5 (1992): 1093–1102.

63. Neubauer and Pratt, "The Second Public Health Revolution"; Allegrante and Green, "Sounding Board"; Crawford, "You Are Dangerous" p. 671; Minkler, "Challenges."

64. U.S. Congress, The Personal Responsibility and Work Opportunity Reconciliation Act, (Washington, D.C., August 1996).

65. Peter Edelman, "The Worst Thing Bill Clinton Has Done," *Atlantic Monthly* 279, no. 3 (March 1997): 43–58.

66. Joanna Weinberg, "Caregiving, Age, and Class in the Skeleton of the Welfare State: 'And Jill Came Tumbling After' . . . " in *Critical Gerontology: Perspectives from Political and Moral Economy,* ed. Meredith Minkler and Carroll Estes (Amityville, N.Y.: Baywood Publishing, 1999); Marc Pilisuk and Meredith Minkler, "Social Support: Economic and Political Considerations," *Social Policy* (Winter 1985): 6–11.

67. Syme, "Rethinking Disease."

68. Robison, "Changing Health Behaviors."

69. Brownell, "Effects of Weight Cycling on Metabolism, Health and Psychological Factors," *Eating Disorders and Obesity: A Comprehensive Handbook,* ed. Kelly D. Brownell and Christopher G. Fairborn (New York: Guilford Press, 1995).

70. Harry Sultz, "Health Policy: If You Don't Know Where You're Going, Any Road Will Take You," *American Journal of Public Health* 81, no. 4 (1991): 418–20.

71. Syme, "Strategies for Health Promotion," *Preventive Medicine* 15 (1986): 492–507.

72. U.S. Department of Health and Human Services, *Preventing Tobacco Use among Young People: A Report of the Surgeon General* (Atlanta, Ga.: U.S. Department of Health and Human Services, Public Health Service, Center for Disease Control and Prevention, National Center for Chronic Disease Prevention and Health Promotion, Office on Smoking and Health, 1994).

73. Syme, "Strategies for Health Promotion."

74. Syme, "Rethinking Disease."

75. B. L. Thompson et al., "Principles of Community Organization and Partnership for Smoking Cessation in the Community Intervention Trial for Smoking Cessation (COMMIT)," *International Quarterly of Community Health Education* 11, no. 3 (1990–1991): 187–203.

76. Farquhar, "Keynote Address."

77. Syme, "Community Participation, Empowerment, and Health: Development of a Wellness Guide for California" (lecture presented at the 1997 California Wellness Foundation/University of California Wellness Lecture Series, Berkeley, Calif., October 1997).

78. Farquhar, "Keynote Address."

79. National Safety Council, *Accident Facts 1997 Edition* (Itasca, Ill.: National Safety Council, 1997).

80. Faith Fitzgerald, "The Tyranny of Health," *NEJM* 331, no. 3 (1994): 196–98.

81. Fitzgerald, "The Tyranny of Health."

82. Becker, "The Tyranny of Health Promotion," p. 20.

83. Becker, "The Tyranny of Health Promotion."

84. Syme, "The Importance of Social Environment for Health and Well-Being," in *Issues and Trends in Health,* ed. Rick Carlson and Brooke Newman (St. Louis, Mo.: C. V. Mosby Co., 1987).

85. World Health Organization, *Report of the Working Group on the Concept and Principles of Health Promotion* (Copenhagen: World Health Organization, 1984).

86. World Health Organization, *Report of the Working Group;* World Health Organization, *Ottawa Charter for Health Promotion.* (Copenhagen: World Health Organization, 1986).

87. Jack Epp, *Achieving Health for All: A Framework for Health Promotion* (Ottawa: National Health and Welfare, Government of Canada, 1986).

88. Ann Pederson, Irving Rootman, and Michel O'Neill, eds., *Health Promotion in Canada* (Toronto: W. B. Saunders, 1994).

89. Pederson, Rootman, and O'Neill, *Health Promotion.*

90. S. Yazdanmehr, "Northwest Territories," in *Health Promotion in Canada,* ed. Ann Pederson, Irving Rootman, and Michel O'Neill (Toronto: W. B. Saunders, 1994), pp. 226–43.

91. Irving Rootman, personal communication from the author, 12 January 1994.

92. Green, "Canadian Health Promotion: An Outsiders View from the Inside," in *Health Promotion in Canada,* ed. Ann Pederson, Irving Rootman, and Michel O'Neill (Toronto: W. B. Saunders, 1994), pp. 314–26.

93. Canadian Public Health Association, *Action Statement for Health Promotion in Canada* (Ottawa: Canadian Public Health Association, 1996).

94. Canadian Public Health Association, *Action Statement.*

BEVERLY OVREBO

Health Promotion and Civil Liberties: The Price of Freedoms and the Price of Health

Everything that needs to be said has already been said. But since no one was listening, it must be said again.—Andre Gide

Ethical debates over health promotion and civil liberties are not new.[1] They comprise an essential part of the American conversation, reflecting unresolved conflicts between the rights of individuals and the rights of communities. Controversies over coercive health measures predate the history of public health, and they are as old as the quarantine of ships suspected of carrying bubonic plague. Concern over civil liberties is as old as the Bill of Rights and is imbedded deep in the American psyche. The constitutionality of coercive health measures was upheld by the landmark Supreme Court decision of *Jacobson v. Massachusetts* (197 U.S. 11, 1905) which, ruling in favor of a compulsory smallpox vaccination law, declared: "[I]n every well-ordered society charged with the duty of conserving the safety of its members the rights of the individual in respect of his liberty may at times, under the pressure of great dangers, be subjected to such restraint, to be enforced by reasonable regulations, as the safety of the general public may demand."[2]

While the debates are old, what is new is the context within which these debates are occurring. The rights and responsibilities of individuals are at issue in managed care, with its emphasis on health promotion and cost containment, driven as it is by market forces and market individualism. How much can managed care require healthful behavior from its clients and employees? Do clients and employees have a duty to act healthfully? Are unhealthful behaviors legitimate grounds for denying health care coverage and employment? Does the requirement to act healthfully violate one's civil liberties? Is it legal or ethical to use unhealthy behavior as the grounds for denying a person work or access to health care?

Also new are the diseases of our age. We have entered the era of emergent and reemergent infectious diseases, for which AIDS is just the forerunner. The AIDS prevention paradigm, which emphasizes health promotion in lieu of traditional public health protections, evolved in part in reaction to perceived threats posed by coercive public health measures for the control of communicable disease.

Protective health measures often come at the price of freedoms. Less restrictive measures, such as health promotion, which focuses on individual behavior change, appear to protect freedoms but are often ineffective in controlling and preventing disease. When is a measure so essential that the restriction of civil liberties is justified? Should measures be promoted because they are least restrictive even if they come at the price of community health? In this paper I will analyze the AIDS prevention paradigm, attempting to draw lessons from AIDS both for managed care and for efforts to prevent disease and promote health in the next century.

Health Promotion and Market Individualism

> The way a society responds to problems of disease reveals its deepest cultural, social and moral values.—Allen Brandt

In keeping with this epigram,[3] the current U.S. response to disease has been driven largely by the shift to managed care, deinvestment in public health, and an emphasis on individual behavior as the primary prevention strategy for promoting health and preventing disease. This response reflects core social values that Barris has termed "market individualism," which is characterized by three closely linked constructs: the supremacy of the free market as a regulatory device, a concomitant belief in individual freedom of choice and personal responsibility, and the elevation of individual satisfaction as the chief goal of public health."[4] It also occurs in a larger social context of widening gaps between rich and poor, escalating rates of poverty and homelessness, epidemics of emergent and reemergent infectious diseases, and declining access to health care.

Managed care carries the promise of containing health costs and increasing the number of years of good health in the overall population through an emphasis on prevention. Its perils are that it is market driven, works best with healthy individuals where the burden of disease is spread over a large population (implicitly excluding persons with greatest need and fewest resources). Managed care reflects the dominant model of justice in American society, what Dan Beauchamp calls "market justice," which emphasizes individual responsibility, minimal collective action, and freedom from collective obligations except to respect other persons' fundamental rights.[5] Public health is in many ways incompatible with managed care. Public health is "not simply the aggregation of individual satisfactions. . . . [I]t is . . . a relation between a population and its environment that does not express itself in individual cases in a meaningful way."[6] Public health is rooted in social justice, guided by the principle that death and disease are collective problems, and all persons are entitled to health protection.[7]

Should managed care, rooted as it is in market justice and market individualism, drive public health? The increasing number of Americans without health insurance is a failure of public health, although it may result in greater economies for managed care. Who pays for the health care of children of undocumented women who have been denied prenatal care? Who cares and pays for homeless people who bear the greatest burdens of diseases both infectious and noninfectious? How do we prevent epidemics of emergent and reemergent disease when those first affected by those epidemics are uninsured and untreated?

In the postwar era in the United States, the focus of public health moved away from health protective measures to an emphasis on health promotion. In part this reflected changing morbidity and mortality patterns, the increasing importance of chronic, noninfectious diseases, and what many hoped would be the total eradication and control of infectious disease. It also resulted from growing recognition among epidemiologists of the complex etiology of many diseases and problems.

One attractive feature of health promotion is that it appears to be minimally restrictive, and because it is individualistic in nature, it suits dominant values. However, as Wallack and Wallerstein have written, health promotion reduces complex problems to a few variables, often ignoring social, cultural, and environmental risk factors, leading to victim blaming.[8] Furthermore, health promotion tends to exclude persons with the problem or most at risk for it in the problem definition and the selection of approaches. Even more, health promotion is most popular among everyone except those with or at risk for the problem. It has the serious unintended consequence of stigmatizing persons with the greatest need and the fewest resources. It tends to benefit vested interests, and is amenable to simple, technological solutions.[9]

The effectiveness of health promotion is contingent on several factors: (1) the risk factor must be causally linked to the disease; (2) the healthy behavior must be causally linked to the risk factor; (3) the healthy behavior must be adopted fully and as planned; and (4) the healthy behavior must be adopted by a population, not just an individual. Syme has noted that the lifestyle approach to understanding and preventing coronary heart disease has proved unsuccessful. The known lifestyle risk factors, which comprise coronary heart disease's web of causation, account for only 40 percent of the coronary heart disease that occurs. Further, as the Multiple Risk Factor Intervention Trial (MRFIT) study showed, it has proven very difficult for people to make changes in their risk behaviors. Finally, "when people do successfully change their risk behaviors, new people continue to enter the 'at risk' population to take their place."[10]

The current "tobacco wars" reflect a more ecological approach to health promotion. The targeted behavior is smoking cigarettes, which has been shown to be a causally significant risk factor in the development of lung cancer. It has also been found that smoking cessation, even after years of heavy smoking, increases the probability of reversing lung damage in populations. The current tobacco wars rely on a broad approach to health promotion, targeting not only "risk takers," but also, "risk makers" (e.g., media and advertisers, the tobacco industry, and retailers). Also targeted are "lateral risk taking" (i.e., passive smoking), and "risky environments," such as restaurants, bars, and public spaces. As a result of these efforts, the rate of cigarette smoking has declined, especially among adult white males, although the use of cigars and other tobacco products has increased. However, as Syme predicted, new people have entered the at-risk population.[11] For example, the rate of cigarette smoking among U.S. high school students increased from 27.5 percent in 1991 to 34.8 percent in 1995.[12] And while lung cancer rates and deaths have decreased among white men, they continue to rise among women and communities of color.

The Case of AIDS

AIDS is arguably the defining disease of the latter part of the twentieth century, challenging public health and the current health care system. AIDS is both an infectious disease and a chronic illness, fatal and pandemic. The United Nations estimates that over 30.6 million persons globally are infected with HIV, with 16,000 new infections occurring each day, and 11.7 million deaths.[13] AIDS has signaled the end of the era of noninfectious disease and brings down the shade on the WHO's goal of eradicating infectious diseases globally. AIDS is now considered to be among the first of many new, emergent diseases. Its appearance coincided with the return of old diseases, once thought to be controlled or eradicated, such as tuberculosis. Tuberculosis is now the number one killer of adults globally and the leading cause of premature mortality in developing countries.[14] AIDS is expected to surpass tuberculosis in this ranking early in the next century, depressing the global economy by as much as 4 percent of the U.S. gross domestic product.[15] AIDS is a disease of social inequity, following the fault lines of society.[16] The increase in AIDS cases has closely followed the epidemic rise of homelessness nationally and globally. AIDS, tuberculosis, homelessness, and many of the major emergent and reemergent diseases tend to coexist in the same persons and populations.

The AIDS Prevention Paradigm

In the early years of the AIDS epidemic, neither the disease's etiology nor effective measures for its control were understood. AIDS proved to be a biological, sociological, and historical puzzle.[17] Government inaction was matched by public apathy, which was followed, in the mid-1980s, by a secondary epidemic: fear of AIDS. Because the disease first affected populations that were highly stigmatized, concern was raised that history would repeat itself, and marginalized populations highly associated with the disease would be blamed and scapegoated. Ethicists and activists rallied against highly restrictive measures that would threaten civil liberties with no guarantees that they would control the epidemic. Specific concern was raised over calls for routine and mandatory HIV testing, contact tracing, mandatory treatment, quarantine, and isolation. In response to these threats to civil liberties, public health and its history of restrictive health-protective measures came under strong scrutiny and attack.

The gay community, at the epicenter of the epidemic when it first hit, played a leadership role in defining AIDS as a disease linked to specific behaviors, not identity; in mobilizing government support and moneys for research and treatment; and in shaping preventive strategies, challenging the model of disease prevention and control used for sexually transmitted diseases (STD) and tuberculosis, in favor of a lifestyle approach.[18] The emergence of the AIDS prevention paradigm can be seen in the famous San Francisco Bathhouse controversy of the mid-1980s. By

1983, cluster studies of AIDS infection provided the Centers for Disease Control (CDC) with evidence that AIDS was a sexually transmissible disease, highly associated with sexual practices of gay men, which practices were most likely to occur in bathhouses.[19] A highly charged public debate ensued over whether or not the public health department should force closure of the bathhouses. Arguments against closure included the lack of definitive proof that AIDS was infectious; the fear that closing the bathhouses would further stigmatize and punish gay men, de facto blaming them for this epidemic; and that the risk factor was not the bathhouses per se, but the behaviors of people within the bathhouses. Public health arguments in favor of closure compared the closing of the bathhouses to John Snow's removal of the Broad Street pump to control the 1854 London cholera epidemic. The bathhouses were allowed to stay open, with the proviso that they become sites for safe sex education. Eventually the bathhouses did close due to market forces, having lost most of their customers.[20]

The victory of the lifestyle model over more restrictive approaches to health protection marked a turning point in public health, testimony to the power that traditionally disenfranchised communities could have in shaping public policy. "Safe sex" as a construct was developed by the gay community, which, as early as 1982, distributed pamphlets describing and rating risky sexual behaviors and advocating the use of condoms. Research shows that safe sex (now termed "safer sex") continues to be widely practiced among the cohort of gay men active in the early years of the AIDS epidemic, who were actively involved in identifying the problem and developing and implementing their own solutions. The power and effectiveness of community participation in health promotion has also been borne out by the successes of the harm reduction movement, which has involved drug users in designing and implementing health education and needle exchange programs.[21]

By involving communities at risk in shaping and implementing programs, safer sex education and harm reduction have protected freedoms. However, because health promotion has been required to carry the burden of prevention, unsupported and uncomplemented by traditional health protective measures, it has come at the price of health. The incidence of HIV/AIDS continues to grow at epidemic rates, having spread to every corner of the globe, depopulating entire segments of the planet, threatening to depopulate the world.

AIDS reveals that traditional approaches to health promotion that rely on lifestyle change, while necessary, are insufficient in the control of infectious disease. Infectious diseases often require aggressive health-protective measures and a global approach to disease control. One only has to travel to a part of the planet where cholera is endemic and there is no sewage system or safe water supply to know how difficult it is to take personal responsibility for one's health. One also learns how easy it is to contract gastrointestinal disease when boiling and filtering one's own water. Environmental protections are restrictive of personal freedoms (e.g., the freedom to have one's own water supply), but if effective, they produce greater freedoms, such as the freedom from infectious disease and the fear of epidemics.

Furthermore, AIDS is a disease of lifestyles and environments, associated with sociocultural risk factors such as poverty and homelessness, oppression and marginalization, inadequate health care and public health infrastructures, sexual exploitation and sex trafficking, war and societal disruption. Just as it has proven very difficult for people to make changes in their risk behaviors for coronary heart disease, so it has been true for risk behaviors for AIDS—and as health educators well know, sexual and addictive behaviors are among the most hard programmed and difficult to change. Finally, as Syme has stated, even when some people have successfully changed their risk behaviors, new people have continued to enter the at-risk population to take their place, (e.g., the epidemic rate of AIDS and HIV among women, adolescents, and communities of color).[22]

In stark contrast to the United States, Cuba addressed AIDS early on as a traditional, infectious epidemic, employing a model of prevention similar to the U.S. tuberculosis control model. When the first cases of AIDS were reported in Cuba in the early 1980s, the Cuban government imposed highly restrictive health-protective measures, isolating all persons with HIV/AIDS and requiring mandatory HIV testing for all persons entering the country. Ten years into the epidemic, the rate of increase of HIV cases was less than 1 percent.[23] The disparate success rates of the Cuban and U.S. AIDS control models prompted Stephen Joseph, director of public health in New York City, to ask if the United States had dealt with AIDS as a civil liberties emergency with public health implications rather than as a public health emergency with civil liberties implications.[24]

AIDS as the New Plague
AIDS has caused a reaching back to the past, a reflection on other epidemics and how societies have handled them. As Fee and Fox have

written, "AIDS has stimulated more interest in history than any other disease in modern times."[25] AIDS has often been called the "new plague," and historic parallels to the scapegoating and persecution of Jews during the Black Death has been cited as a warning against the threats to health and freedoms of broadly restrictive public health measures.[26]

History is replete with examples of public health measures, which were both discriminatory and ineffective.[27] Failed and oppressive public health efforts to control plague when it first emerged in the Western Hemisphere are a case in point. Bubonic plague entered the United States in San Francisco in 1900. In that same year, San Francisco's Department of Public Health quarantined Chinatown and its 25,000 residents because of one case of bubonic plague contracted by a Chinese man, Chick Gin. Homes were forcibly inspected, thousands of Chinese people were incarcerated at Angel Island, and in May 1900, the city came within hours of burning down Chinatown, with the residents inside. In spite of these efforts, plague spread, and by 1904 a total of 120 people, all Chinese, had contracted the disease, 100 of whom died.[28]

Less often cited is the quick and positive turnaround in the actions and policies of public health, and the positive role understanding the disease's etiology played in changing the attitudes of the public and civil authorities. This turn was evidenced in the second San Francisco plague outbreak, which erupted after the earthquake of 1906. Over a period of eighteen months, 160 persons contracted the disease (almost none of them Chinese), seventy-eight of whom died. By this time, however, bubonic plague as a vector-borne disease associated with rats was finally understood, and the San Francisco plague epidemic was halted through aggressive rodent control. No attacks on the Chinese or Chinatown occurred.[29] These preventive measures were incorporated into the public health infrastructure and have allowed San Francisco to live free from plaque for ninety years.

Reflecting on the parallels that have been drawn between AIDS and the plague, Fee and Fox have written,

> Both the alarmists and the advocates of equanimity agreed that AIDS was a contemporary plague. They shared the belief that history was pertinent to understanding the epidemic and that the events in the past that were most pertinent were those surrounding sudden, time-limited outbreaks of infection. . . . Many people were unwilling to believe that a disease that had emerged (it seemed) so suddenly, and appeared to be invariably fatal, was either deeply rooted in the past or likely to become part of the human condition for the foreseeable future.[30]

They go on to write:

Because the history of visitations of plagues was the only history that appeared relevant to the new epidemic, most people ignored the alternative historical models that were available. For example, most of those who used historical analogies avoided the most pertinent aspects of the histories of venereal disease and tuberculosis. . .[31]

AIDS: The Great Exception?

There is currently a reexamination of the U.S. AIDS response and renewed advocacy for the adoption of traditional models of disease prevention and control, such as those used with tuberculosis, and STDs, which combine health promotion and health protections. As Lee Reichman, director of the National Tuberculosis Center has stated,

Traditional public health is absolutely effective at controlling infectious disease. It should have been applied to AIDS from the start, and it wasn't. Long before there was AIDS, there were other sexually transmitted diseases, and you had partner notification and testing and reporting. This was routine public health at its finest, and this is the way STDs were controlled.[32]

There is no guarantee, however, that more traditional public health measures will work or would have worked to control AIDS, and the threats these measures pose to civil liberties are very real. It is also unlikely that the Cuban model could have successfully been imposed on U.S. society. As many have suggested, a broadly restrictive approach to AIDS may have driven the disease further underground and led to massive scapegoating and discrimination against persons associated with the disease.[33] Furthermore, Cuba is an island nation with a relatively small population and broad and effective police powers. Finally, as Hamm points out, Cuba had a higher literacy rate and universal health care, both of which are highly associated with positive health outcomes in a society.[34]

Researchers now say, "the development of a safe and inexpensive HIV vaccine is the only hope of taming the global AIDS epidemic."[35] Assuming a safe and effective HIV vaccine can be developed, HIV vaccination will have to be deployed globally with the cooperation of all nations. At best it would be a slow cure. The global smallpox eradication program took 20 years to implement. To succeed, such a program would have to be compulsory, undoubtedly facing court challenges to its constitutionality, again testing the rationale for treating community rights as superior to individual rights.[36]

The U.S. AIDS response has been driven by market individualism and market justice. AIDS is often measured in market terms—the cost-benefits of care and treatment, the market opportunities AIDS provides (what is now termed the AIDS industry). Thus far AIDS has accommodated itself well to the marketplace. However, it is predicted that by 2005 AIDS will depress the global economy by as much as 4 percent of the U.S. gross domestic product.[37] AIDS is becoming a public health and market disaster.

AIDS not only follows the fault lines of society, but it reveals society's faults—deep-seated social inequity, discrimination against persons with disease and those most at risk for disease, an emphasis on personal responsibility for health, a reliance on tertiary treatment over primary prevention, a distrust of the government's ability to prevent and control disease, and the lack of a global vision of disease control.

As the threat AIDS poses to the global marketplace becomes more evident and as it becomes clearer that AIDS is a disease predominantly affecting people held in the lowest regard, concern over civil liberties may be overridden by a concern for the public's safety. Underlying all civil liberties debates are questions of whose civil liberties are at stake and whose health is at risk.

This shift in public attitudes was in evidence in the isolation and quarantine of Kikwit, Zaire, in May 1995 during an outbreak of Ebola. For a period of two weeks, no one was allowed to enter or leave this city of 400,000 people. Homes were forcibly inspected for cases and fatalities, and family members were arrested for nursing persons with Ebola, or for burying the dead. Protest was raised in Kikwit and among some Zairians over the harsh restrictions and the danger imposed on all residents of the city, but international concern focused on the threat of spread of Ebola to the rest of the planet. Harsh, restrictive measures worked to stop the epidemic.[38] One must question whether a similar response would have been tolerated in the United States.

Government has a duty to protect the freedoms of individuals and a duty to protect the public's health. As the health, social, and economic costs of AIDS escalate, it is clear that the focus of protecting civil liberties has come at the price of freedoms and the price of health. The AIDS response has been ineffective, and victim blaming in its most extreme form, with the duty to protect the public's health falling on individuals who are increasingly those members of societies with the fewest resources and power. The threats AIDS poses to civil liberties are real. As the health and social costs of AIDS grow and it becomes more evident that AIDS is a disease of poverty and disenfranchisement, the calls for restrictive measures are certain to increase. AIDS is, and will remain, both a public health and a civil liberties emergency.

Conclusion

The price of freedom is eternal vigilance.—Thomas Jefferson

Conflicts between health promotion and civil liberties will never be fully resolved. In each era, these conflicts must be resolved.

That managed care is leaning hard on health promotion is suggested by a 1993 position paper by the California Conference of Local Directors of Health Educators: "The utility of health promotion and health-education programs to postpone and prevent catastrophic illness cannot be ignored or underestimated if improvement in both the public health's status and the State's fiscal health is the desired outcome of health care reform."[39]

In an era of emergent and reemergent disease, the strategies of health promotion and curative medicine are necessary but not sufficient to protect the public's health. AIDS instructs that diseases must be addressed at the level of root causes, and the basic infrastructures and tools of public health must be preserved and strengthened. Further, as the Tobacco Wars have illustrated, health promotion is most effective when it targets riskmakers as well as risktakers. Be it with carrots or sticks, imposing a duty on individuals to act healthfully neither works nor is least restrictive. As Minkler and others have written, health promotion is most effective and ethical when it starts where people are, and involves target populations in the definition of the problem and selection of approaches.[40]

Managed care with its emphases on market solutions and individual responsibility has failed to recognize inherent conflicts between market individualism and public health: "How the market puts our health at risk, how individual choices are mediated by individual and social conditions, and how the welfare of the community can diverge from the welfare of the individual."[41]

The managed care strategy of containing costs through coercive health promotion and curative treatments is set to exacerbate the current ills of the health care system, decreasing access to care, depressing health outcomes, and shifting blame for disease and disability to the poor and disenfranchised. As Jencks has stated, "Even in the world's most commercialized society, blame is still free. That means there is still plenty for everyone."[42]

Coercive health promotion is social control at its most insidious, reflecting the new healthism, the need to blame someone, and the pervasive view that people who behave unhealthfully are legitimate targets of disapproval and punishment. The harm reduction movement offers a socially just alternative, working with at-risk populations and directly confronting the need to scapegoat, taking the stance that "inflicting harm on drug users is not a legitimate way to express our disapproval of their behavior."[43]

In this new era of disease, a health care system is required that addresses and is responsive to social inequity; that has the tools and means to prevent and control infectious disease; and that is guided by the larger vision, values, and structure of public health. A good start is for managed care to adopt L. Naake's recommendation to the President's Health Care Task Force, that a specific percentage of total health expenditures be set aside for public health.[44] Managed care must be guided by the precepts of public health, not market individualism, to endeavor to "do no harm" and leave no harm in its wake.

Market individualism has made public health unthinkable.[45] The prospect of short-term profits is not worth the price. As AIDS instructs, it comes at the price of freedoms and the price of health.

NOTES

1. This chapter is based on a presentation given at the Hastings Center Meetings on Health Promotion and Disease Prevention: Ethical and Social Dilemmas in Los Angeles (December 11, 1997) and San Francisco (December 12, 1997). The epigram was cited in Willard Gaylin, Ira Glasser, Steven Marcus, and David J. Rothman, *Doing Good: The Limits of Benevolence* (New York: Pantheon Books, 1978), p. 168.

2. Josephine Gittler, "Controlling Resurgent Tuberculosis: Public Health Agencies, Public Policy, and Law," *Journal of Health Politics, Policy and Law* 19, no. 1 (1994): 107–47.

3. Allen Brandt, "AIDS: From Social History to Social Policy," in *AIDS: The Burdens of History,* eds. E. Fee and D. Fox, Berkeley, Calif.: University of California Press, 1988, pp. 147–171, at 147.

4. Scott Barris, "The Invisibility of Public Health: Population-Level Measures in a Politics of Market Individualism," *American Journal of Public Health* 87, no. 10 (1997): 1607–10.

5. Dan E. Beauchamp, "Public Health as Social Justice," *Inquiry* 13 (March 1976): 3–13.

6. Barris, "The Invisibility of Public Health," p. 1609.

7. Beauchamp, "Public Health as Social Justice."

8. Larry Wallack and Nina Wallerstein, "Health Education and Prevention, Designing Community Initiatives," *International Quarterly of Community Health Education* 7, no. 4 (1986–87): 319–42.

9. Wallack and Wallerstein, "Health Education and Prevention," p. 325.

10. S. Leonard Syme, "Rethinking Disease: Where Do We Go from Here," *Annals of Epidemiology* 6, no. 5 (1996): 463–68, at 463.

11. S. Syme, "Rethinking Disease."

12. Centers for Disease Control and Prevention, "Tobacco Use and Usual Source of Cigarettes among High School Students—United States, 1995," *Morbidity and Mortality Weekly Report* (May 24, 1996).

13. Chronicle News Service, "UN Doubles Estimate of New HIV Cases," *San Francisco Chronicle* (November 26, 1997), p. A2.

14. Kevin M. DeCock, "Tuberculosis Control in Resource-Poor Settings with High Rates of HIV Infection," *American Journal of Public Health* 86, no. 8 (1996): 1071–73.

15. Zena Stein and Mervyn Susser, "AIDS: An Update on Global Dynamics," *American Journal of Public Health* 87, no. 6 (1997): 901–04.

16. Mary Catherine Bateson and Richard Goldsby, *Thinking AIDS: The Social Response to the Biological Threat* (Reading, Mass: Addison-Wesley Publishing Co., Inc., 1988).

17. Elizabeth Fee, "Health Education: Looking Backward, Looking Forward." (Lecture given at San Francisco State University, August 1994).

18. Dennis Altman, "Legitimation through Disaster: AIDS and the Gay Movement," *AIDS: The Burdens of History,* ed. Elizabeth Fee and Daniel Fox (Berkeley, Calif: University of California Press, 1988), pp. 310–15.

19. Gerald M. Oppenheimer, "Causes, Cases and Cohorts: The Role of Epidemiology in the Historical Construction of AIDS," *AIDS: The Making of a Chronic Disease,* ed. Elizabeth Fee and Daniel Fox (Berkeley, Calif.: University of California Press, 1992), pp. 49–83.

20. Randy Shilts, *And the Band Played On: Politics, People and the AIDS Epidemic* (New York: St. Martins Press, 1987).

21. Leonard H. Glantz and Wendy K. Mariner, "Needle Exchange Programs and the Law—Time for a Change," *American Journal of Public Health* 86, no. 8 (1996): 1077–79.

22. Syme, "Rethinking Disease."

23. Lyta Hamm, "Archipelago Lessons: AIDS in the Islands—A Comparative Study of Cuba, Haiti and Hawaii," *Interciencia* 86, no. 8 (1993): 184–89.

24. Stephen Joseph, cited in Josephine Gittler, "Controlling Resurgent Tuberculosis." Public Health Agencies, Public Policy, and Law," *Journal of Health Politics, Policy and Law* 19, no. 1 (1994): 107–47.

25. Fee and Fox, "Introduction: AIDS, Public Policy, and Historical Inquiry," in *AIDS: The Burdens of History,* pp. 1–11.

26. David F. Musto, "Quarantine and the Problem of AIDS," in *AIDS: The Burdens of History,* pp. 67–85.

27. Brandt, "AIDS: From Social History to Social Policy," pp. 147–71; Musto, "Quarantine and the Problem of AIDS," pp. 67–85; Sylvia Tesh, *Hidden*

Arguments (New Brunswick, NJ: Rutgers University Press, 1988); Allen Kraut, *Silent Travelers: Genes, Germs and the Immigrant Menace* (New York: Basic Books, 1994); William McNeill, *Plagues and Peoples* (Garden City, NY: Doubleday Books, 1976).

28. Kraut, *Silent Travelers.*

29. Kraut, *Silent Travelers.*

30. Fee and Fox, "Introduction: The Contemporary Historiography of AIDS," in *AIDS: The Making of a Chronic Disease,* pp. 1–22, at 1.

31. Fee and Fox, "Introduction: The Contemporary Historiography of AIDS," pp. 3–4.

32. Lee Riechman, cited in Chandler Burr, "The AIDS Exception: Privacy vs. Public Health," *Atlantic Monthly* (June 1997): 57–67, at 66.

33. Musto, "Quarantine and the Problem of AIDS," pp. 67–85.

34. Lyta Hamm, "Archipelago Lessons."

35. Seth Berkeley, "The International AIDS Vaccine Initiative," *Journal of the International Association of Physicians in AIDS* 3, no. 11 (1997), p. 30.

36. Josephine Gittler, "Controlling Resurgent Tuberculosis," p. 123.

37. Stein and Susser, "AIDS."

38. Laurie Garrett, "Plague Warriors," *Vanity Fair* (August 1995): 85–93, 156–61.

39. California Conference of Local Directors of Health Education, *The Role of Health Promotion/Health Education in a Managed Care Setting,* p. 1.

40. Meredith Minkler and Cheri Pies, "Ethical Issues in Community Organizing and Community Participation" in *Community Organizing and Community Building for Health,* ed. Meredith Minkler (New Brunswick, NJ: Rutgers University Press, 1997), pp. 120–38; Ann Robertson and Meredith Minkler, "New Health Promotion: A Critical Examination," *Health Education Quarterly* 21, no. 3 (1994): 295–312.

41. Barris, "The Invisibility of Public Health," p. 1610.

42. Christopher Jencks, "The Truth about the Homeless," *New York Review of Books* (April 21, 1994), p. 27.

43. Glantz and Mariner, "Needle Exchange Programs and the Law," p. 1078.

44. L. Naake, Statement on Behalf of the National Association of Counties before the President's Health Task Force (March 1993), cited in California Conference of Local Directors of Health Education, *The Role of Health Promotion/Health Education in a Managed Care Setting,* p. 11.

45. Barris, "The Invisibility of Public Health."

Helen Halpin Schauffler

The Credibility of Claims for the Economic Benefits of Health Promotion

Three claims are often made about the economic benefits of health promotion:

1. Health promotion provides a return on its investment through medical care cost savings.
2. Health maintenance organizations (HMOs) have an economic incentive to promote the health of their members.
3. Health promotion is cost-effective.

In this article I will review the scientific evidence and political motivations behind each of these economic claims. In addition, to the extent that there are discrepancies between the scientific evidence and the claims, I will discuss the ethical dilemmas that these discrepancies pose for health promotion advocates and will conclude with a discussion of how advocates could better frame their arguments for increasing spending on health promotion in light of the available scientific evidence on the economic benefits. Scientific evidence is defined as research based on randomized control trials (RCT) or observational studies that estimate costs, effectiveness, and economic benefits measured in terms of medical care cost savings per dollar spent on health promotion interventions. Cost-benefit ratios based on case-control designs or hypothetical projections using secondary data sources do not qualify as meeting scientific standards of evidence.

Economic Claims of Medical Care Cost Savings

Claims that health-promotion interventions are cost savings to the medical care system have been made by the top administrators of federal public health agencies; public health leaders in academia; health promotion advocates at national, state, and local levels; and providers of health-promotion interventions.[1] Their claim is that health promotion will yield a return on its investment, such that spending on health promotion will result in decreased health services utilization and reduced medical care costs.

There is no question that health-promotion advocates strongly believe, and promote the belief, that health promotion saves medical care dollars. In fact, this precise claim was at the foundation of the materials produced and the arguments made by public health advocates during the health care reform debates of the 103rd Congress (1993–1994). The Centers for Disease Control and Prevention (CDC) published and widely distributed a 1993 monograph titled *An Ounce of Prevention: What Are the Returns?*[2] The Department of Health and Human Services (DHHS) similarly published and distributed a 1994 monograph titled *For a Healthy Nation: Returns on Investment in Public Health.*[3] The Partnership for Prevention, a broad-based coalition in Washington, D.C., published a 1994 monograph that was distributed to members of the U.S. Congress titled *Prevention: Benefits, Costs, and Savings.*[4] In every case, health promotion was sold and marketed as cost saving. Claims that investments in health promotion will reduce medical care costs have become the mantras of public health advocates seeking to increase both public and private spending on health promotion. What is the credibility of these economic claims of medical cost savings?

In preparing its 1993 monograph, CDC reviewed more than 3,200 scientific articles published between 1979 and 1990 on the effectiveness and cost-effectiveness of prevention strategies and programs.[5] They reported only five examples of medical cost savings that fell into two broad areas: immunizations and prenatal care (Table 1).

The interventions cited as cost saving included the pneumococcal vaccine, which was estimated in 1990 to save $141 per person over the age of 50 who receives it;[6] the measles, mumps, and rubella (MMR) vaccine for children, which was estimated in 1985 to save $14 for every dollar spent;[7] prenatal care for low-income, poorly educated women, which was estimated in 1985 to save $3.40 in medical care during the first year of life for every dollar spent;[8] management of diabetes in early pregnancy, which was estimated in 1992 to save $5.19 for every dollar spent;[9] and smoking cessation for pregnant women, which was estimated in 1990 to save $6 in neonatal intensive care and long-term care costs for every dollar spent.[10] These five examples were the total sum of the evidence CDC presented in 1993 that prevention provides an economic return on its investment.[11]

Table 1. Claims of Medical Cost Savings by Public Health Leaders during the Health Care Reform Debates of the 103rd Congress (1993–1994)

Author	Year	Intervention	Study Population	Claimed Medical Cost Savings per Dollar Spent	Research Design
C B Gable et al.	1990	Pneumococcal vaccine	Adults 65 years and older	$141/person	Case-Control
C C White et al.	1985	Measles, mumps, rubella vaccine	Birth cohort through age 30	$14.00	Hypothetical projection
Prenatal Care					
Institute of Medicine	1985	Prenatal care	Low-income, poorly educated, pregnant women	$3.40	Hypothetical projection
R Scheffler et al.	1992	Management of diabetes	Pregnant women with diabetes	$5.19	Case-Control
J S Marks et al.	1990	Smoking cessation	Pregnant women	$6.00	Hypothetical projection
Battelle report	1994	Childhood immunizations	Children	$8.80	Hypothetical projection
Population Health					
Battelle report	1994	Prevent heart disease, stroke, motor vehicle injuries, low birthweight, and gunshot wounds	US population	$68.9 billion over 6 years	Hypothetical projection

None of the above cost-benefit ratios cited by CDC was based on research designed to meet the criteria established for scientific evidence. The research estimating cost savings for the pneumococcal vaccine was based on a case-control study that used estimates from a retrospective cohort study on vaccination and age-sex matched persons who had not been vaccinated.[12] The study published on the costs and benefits of the MMR vaccine for children was based on comparison with a hypothetical situation using estimates from secondary sources, assuming there had not been an immunization program.[13] The estimate of cost-savings for prenatal care for low-income, poorly educated women was based on hypothetical projections using secondary data sources.[14] The research estimating cost-savings for the management of diabetes in pregnancy was a retrospective, case-control study.[15] The research estimating cost-savings for smoking cessation for pregnant women was based on projected costs and benefits from secondary sources using theoretical assumptions.[16]

In 1994, the DHHS conducted its own review of the evidence of cost savings for prevention and public health interventions and added only one more intervention to CDC's list: complete childhood immunizations, which were estimated in 1990 to save $8.80 in medical costs attributable to low birthweight infants for every dollar spent.[17] However, the source of DHHS's evidence on cost savings from childhood immunizations was a 1994 Battelle report that was never published in a peer-reviewed journal.[18]

The Partnership for Prevention, in their 1994 monograph on the costs, benefits, and savings of prevention, cited the same examples of cost-savings as CDC and DHHS, including the pneumococcal vaccine for people over fifty, childhood immunizations, and prenatal care for low-income, poorly educated women, adding no new evidence to support their claim of cost savings.[19]

In reviewing more than three hundred published scientific articles that analyzed the costs and benefits of health-promotion strategies and programs published in peer-reviewed journals for the fifteen-year period from 1982 through 1997, nine studies were found to have met the standards of scientific evidence (Table 2). These interventions fall into three areas:

1. Prenatal care for pregnant women addressing smoking cessation and nutrition.

Table 2. Additional Evidence of Medical Care Cost Savings from Prevention Interventions, 1982–1997

Author	Year	Intervention	Study Population	Research Design	Medical Cost Savings per Dollar Spent
Immunizations					
K L Nichols et al.	1994	Influenza vaccine	Men and women over age 64	Observational study	$1.64
K L Nichols et al.	1995	Influenza vaccine	Working adults age 18–64	Controlled trial	$1.56
Prenatal Care					
D H Ershoff et al.	1983	Nutrition counseling and smoking cessation	Pregnant women smokers in an HMO	Observational study	$2.00
B Devaney et al.	1992	WIC	Pregnant women on Medicaid	Observational study	$1.77–$3.13
P A Buescher et al.	1993	WIC	Pregnant women on Medicaid	Observational study	$2.91
Health Education					
W Neresian et al.	1982	Diabetes education	Men and women with diabetes	Observational study	$2.95
C E Lewis et al.	1984	Asthma education	Children with diabetes, ages 7–12, in an HMO	Controlled trial	$1.44
D M Vickery et al.	1983	Self-care education	Households in an HMO	Controlled trial	$2.41–$3.43

2. Health education programs for persons with chronic conditions and self-care for minor complaints.
3. Prevention of infectious disease.

Prenatal Care for Smoking Cessation and Nutrition

Two studies were identified to estimate the costs and benefits of the Special Supplemental Food Program for Women, Infants and Children (WIC). WIC provides supplemental food, nutrition and health education, and social services referrals to pregnant, breast-feeding, and post-partum women and their infants and young children who are low-income and at nutritional risk.[20] Two observational studies of women who received Medicaid and who did and did not participate in the WIC program found that women who participated in WIC had a lower rate of low-birthweight babies compared with non-participants.[21] One study on the effects of prenatal WIC participation and the use of prenatal care on Medicaid costs and birth outcomes in five states estimated that during the first 60 days following birth, between $1.77 and $3.13 was saved in medical costs to Medicaid for every dollar spent.[22] The other study estimated medical cost savings to Medicaid of $2.91 for every dollar spent on WIC services.[23] A meta analysis and a comprehensive review of prenatal WIC studies confirm these estimated medical cost savings to the Medicaid program.[24]

Two other prevention interventions that provided health education, specifically addressing smoking and nutrition to pregnant women as part of prenatal care, provide evidence of medical care cost savings. One study that provided a smoking cessation program to pregnant smokers was estimated in 1991 to save between $6.72 and $17.18 per dollar spent. This study was a prospective, randomized, control group, pretest/posttest design conducted from 1986 to 1991 on 814 pregnant smokers who entered prenatal care prior to thirty-two weeks.[25]

The other intervention was a prenatal nutrition and smoking cessation program that was estimated to save two dollars in medical costs per dollar spent as a result of fewer low-birthweight babies.[26] The study, which used a quasi-experimental research design, was a non-randomized, observational study that followed an experimental (N = 57) and control (N = 72) group of women who were smokers at the time of pregnancy testing. The experimental group was enrolled in an eight-week smoking cessation program that included a home correspondence format, meeting with a health educator, and participation in two forty-five-minute, individual nutrition counseling sessions. Women in the control group received standard prenatal care. The women were followed until two months postpartum. Outcomes tracked included changes in health behaviors, birth outcomes (low birthweight), and medical costs per delivery.[27]

Another study on the cost and benefits of smoking cessation for pregnant women was identified, but it was based on a decision-tree model using secondary sources for estimates of the effectiveness of smoking cessation for pregnant women and other assumptions about the costs of the intervention, quit rates, and medical care costs averted.[28]

Health Education

Two studies were identified that provided evidence on the costs and benefits of health education programs to manage chronic disease.[29] One was a health education program for children with asthma, ages seven to twelve that was estimated to save $180 per child per year through reductions in emergency room visits and hospitalizations, or $1.44 saved in one year for every dollar spent.[30] This study was an RCT of Asthma Care Training for kids. The number of emergency room visits and days of hospitalization were reduced significantly more in the experimental (N = 48) compared with the control (N = 28) group.[31]

A diabetes education program was estimated to save $292 per participant, or $2.95 saved in medical costs per dollar spent.[32] The study was a prospective, observational study over a three-year period. A total of 461 persons with diabetes completed classes in self-monitoring, insulin regulation, nutrition education, foot care, and other topics at twenty-six education sites. Changes in hospitalizations one year prior to participation and twelve months following were used to estimate cost savings.[33]

One study was identified that provided evidence on the medical cost savings associated with reduced total medical visits and minor illness visits from a self-care education intervention.[34] This study was an RCT of 1,625 households to determine the intervention's effect on ambulatory care utilization in an HMO. The educational intervention consisted of written materials and individual counseling on self-care for minor illnesses. The intervention was associated with a decrease in total ambulatory visits and a decrease in utilization for minor illnesses that produced estimated medical cost savings in 1983 ranging from $2.41 to $3.43 per dollar spent.[35]

Immunizations

Only one additional study estimating medical cost savings for the pneumococcal vaccine among the elderly was identified, but it was based on a Markov decision-tree model following two hypothetical cohorts, one vaccinated and the other not.[36] Another study on medical cost-savings associated with childhood vaccinations against chicken pox was identified, but it was based on a decision-analysis model estimating incidence and costs from secondary data sources.[37]

The only immunization for which scientific evidence on medical cost-savings could be identified is the influenza vaccine.[38] One study of the effectiveness of the influenza vaccine on healthy, working adults estimated cost savings in 1994 of $5.99 per person, or $1.56 saved in medical care costs associated with physician office visits for upper respiratory infections for every dollar spent.[39] This study was a randomized, double-blind, placebo-controlled trial with a total of 849 subjects. A second study on the effectiveness of the influenza vaccine in the elderly was a serial, observational cohort study with internal controls. The influenza vaccine was associated with significant reductions in hospitalization costs for elderly persons. The direct savings in medical costs attributable to the influenza vaccine was $117 for each elderly person immunized, or approximately $1.64 per dollar spent.[40]

Preventive Screening

No scientific evidence of medical care cost savings was identified for any preventive screening intervention for the early detection of disease.

The Ethical Dilemma for Claims of Medical Care Cost Savings

In 1993 and 1994, health-promotion advocates could not point to a single, prospective observational research study or RCT that provided scientific evidence that any health promotion intervention saved more in medical care expenditures than it cost. A recent review of the scientific evidence of medical care cost savings associated with health promotion interventions identified documented cost savings from the influenza vaccine, selected prenatal smoking cessation and nutrition programs, and selected health education programs for children with asthma, persons with diabetes, and self-care for minor complaints. This handful of prevention interventions are the only ones for which there is any documentation of medical care cost savings meeting scientific standards of evidence.

Why do health promotion advocates make such bold statements about the medical cost savings from health promotion when the empirical evidence is limited to only a few examples that fall within very narrowly defined interventions? The primary reason is political. Over the last five years, when public policy priorities have focused on eliminating the federal budget deficit, limiting the role of government, and controlling medical care costs, and when private health care policy has been dominated by large, consolidated, competing, for-profit managed care corporations, the only way to get attention at the policy table is to argue loudly and consistently that your programs will save money—even when there is little evidence that most of them will.

The discrepancy between the scientific evidence and the medical cost-saving claims raises a fundamental ethical dilemma for health promotion advocates. If for the vast majority of health promotion and disease prevention interventions there is no demonstrated evidence that they will reduce medical care costs, what justifications do health promotion advocates give for continuing to make these claims? Some might argue that if the "ends" translate into increased resources for health promotion programs, as well as increased health insurance coverage for preventive services, then "the ends justify the means." Others might argue that "everyone else is doing it," so that unless health promotion also makes medical care cost-saving claims, they will get little or nothing more when the resource pies are divided.

Are health promotion advocates willing to compromise their integrity in the name of improving the public's health? What happens when those who make "investments" in prevention discover that the promised medical care cost savings were greatly exaggerated or simply not true?

Claims that HMOs Have an Incentive to Promote Health

The claim that HMOs have an economic incentive to promote the health of their members is based on the fact that capitated managed care plans must deliver a comprehensive set of health care services to their members within a fixed budget. Given finite resources, this argument suggests that it is in the economic interests of HMOs to invest in those health promotion interventions that provide immediate or short-term returns (less than one to two years) measured by reduced health services utilization and associated health care costs. This argument is based on the fundamental belief that spending on health promotion will save HMOs money. But as was previously established, we know of very few health promotion interventions for which there is any scientific evidence of medical care cost savings.

Part of the lore that managed care has an incentive to promote the health of their members comes from some of the earliest and most well-known HMOs in the United States, which had, as part of their original mission, a core value of health promotion. These HMOs included Kaiser Permanente, Group Health Cooperative of Pudget Sound, and Harvard Community Health Plan. All of these HMOs were staff or group model HMOs—their physicians were on salary, they were founded as nonprofit organizations with a goal to serve the community, and they were for many years the only HMOs operating in their service areas. But in the 1990s most of these HMOs are not what they were in the 1970s, and most HMOs created since 1980 do not in any way resemble the original HMOs in structure, mission, or in the financial incentives they face.[41]

Most of the growth in HMOs in the United States over the last ten to fifteen years has been in what are called independent practice association (IPA) or network model HMOs in which the HMO itself does not provide any direct services, but instead contracts with IPAs, medical groups, individual doctors, and hospitals to provide medical care to enrollees. The majority of HMOs in the United States in 1998 are for-profit organizations, many of which operate in very competitive environments based on price and perceived quality.[42] There is little incentive to provide any services beyond those that the purchasers demand, for which performance is being tracked as part of quality assurance, or which are offered as part of a competitive marketing strategy.

Evidence from California suggests that nearly all HMOs offer health promotion programs to their members, but fewer than half of enrollees are aware of their availability, and only about 2 percent of enrollees participate in any health promotion program offered by their plan in any given year.[43] Data from a 1996 survey of all HMOs in California suggest that for the majority of HMOs, health promotion programs are not offered with the expectation that they will reduce costs, but instead are provided primarily as a marketing device. Less than one-third of California HMOs report that they assess the impact of the health promotion programs they offer on member health status, health services utilization, or health care costs. Instead, HMOs view health promotion programs as crucial to maintaining their position in the market and as a way to differentiate their plan from competitors.[44]

However, HMOs are most likely to offer health promotion programs where there is scientific evidence of short-term cost savings—prenatal nutrition, smoking cessation, and immunizations.[45] Health promotion interventions for which there is not documented evidence of cost savings within one year are much less likely to be offered. Benefits that would accrue to an HMO in a time frame longer than one year may not be realized, given that approximately 15 percent of HMO members change health plans every year.

In fact, the opposite of the claim that HMOs have an economic incentive to promote the health of their members may be true in the most competitive markets. Market forces operating under managed competition may reduce or eliminate incentives HMOs have to offer health promotion services, since most are not cost saving, but require additional resources to implement. Pressures to lower capitation rates and squeeze budgets may eventually force HMOs to drop what little health promotion they presently offer. In a competitive marketplace, this particular economic claim may get turned completely on its head.

The Ethical Dilemma for Claims that HMOs Have an Economic Incentive to Promote the Health of Their Members

Given the evidence and pressures in the marketplace, why do HMOs claim and health promotion advocates advance the notion that HMOs have an incentive to promote health? This claim, too, has political utility. Perhaps as a society we can feel better about pushing most insured people into managed care, for better or worse, if we believe that HMOs have an incentive to care about their health. HMOs are economically motivated to make claims about how much they want to keep us well, particularly if this claim is attractive to potential members and purchasers who may be persuaded to choose or offer a plan based on such claims.

To the HMO the financial bottom line is the total number of members enrolled in their plan—anything HMOs can do to increase enrollment translates into additional revenues. However, consumers and purchasers must be aware, as is true for all commercial products, that there may not always be truth in advertising.

Evidence from California suggests that purchasers can, through their contracts with HMOs, force managed care plans to offer, promote, and measure performance; set performance targets; and be held financially at risk for not meeting negotiated targets for health promotion.[46] An example of this approach is the quality performance measure based on the percentage of smokers in an HMO who were counseled to quit smoking at their last medical care visit. The Pacific Business Group on Health (PBGH) requires HMOs to improve their performance on this and other measures every year, and if an HMO fails to meet their negotiated target performance level, it must pay PBGH back an amount equal to the percentage of premium placed at risk for meeting that target.[47] The question then becomes, for what health promotion and other services should purchasers require performance guarantees? HMO efforts to establish the necessary data systems to track performance and to implement interventions to improve performance come at a price. Requiring HMOs to absorb new costs without an increase in capitated premiums means that expenditures on something else must be decreased. Capitation is a zero sum game.

Claims that Health Promotion Is Cost-Effective

The claim that spending on health promotion interventions are cost-effective by improving health suggests that the valued outcome is not monetary savings, but improved health status. There is a tremendous amount of evidence on the efficacy and effectiveness of health promotion interventions. For example, it has been demonstrated that quitting smoking improves health, and health promotion interventions such as physician advice to quit, nicotine replacement therapy, and behavioral programs have all been demonstrated to be effective in helping people to quit smoking. Recently, the Agency for Health Care Policy Research (AHCPR) published a summary of the evidence on the effectiveness of smoking cessation interventions.[48]

Dozens of other clinical preventive services have been demonstrated to improve health.[49] For example, it has been demonstrated that many immunizations are effective in preventing infectious diseases; many preventive screening interventions are effective at detecting disease early and reducing associated morbidity and mortality; and many health education and preventive counseling interventions have reduced health risks and prevent future disease and premature death. The scientific evidence on the efficacy and effectiveness of clinical preventive services was documented exhaustively in the U.S. Preventive Services Task Force report, "Guide to Clinical Prevention Services," first published in 1989 and updated in 1996.[50]

Other health promotion and public health interventions have also been demonstrated to be effective in promoting the health of the population. Environmental protections have been demonstrated to be effective in reducing disease, for example, fluoride in the water supply to prevent tooth decay.[51] Injury prevention interventions have also been demonstrated to be effective in reducing disability and saving lives. Examples include the use of seat belts, bicycle helmets, and infant car seats; smoke detectors in homes; and occupational safety and health codes to protect workers on the job.[52] In sum, the evidence is overwhelming that many health promotion interventions are effective in promoting and improving the public's health.

There is also a growing body of evidence that suggests that many health promotion interventions are relatively cost-effective.[53] Cost-effectiveness tells us how much it costs to achieve a particular health outcome, for example, how much we have to spend for each life-year gained, quality life-year gained, life saved, or disease prevented. Cost-effectiveness ratios have been estimated for pap smears and mammograms, smoking cessation and exercise programs, cholesterol and blood pressure reduction and control programs, and injury prevention programs, to name a few.

However, one problem with using estimates of cost-effectiveness to compare the value of different health promotion interventions as the basis for making resource allocation decisions is that there is no standard methodology for estimating either costs or health benefits.[54] Cost-effectiveness estimates have limited value unless the relative cost-effectiveness of one intervention can be compared with another. If different methods are used to estimate costs and/or benefits, it is difficult, if not impossible, to make comparisons. The lack of a common set of techniques in cost-effectiveness analysis produces widely variable, contradictory, and often incomparable results.[55] For example, breast cancer screening has been estimated to cost from $3,000 to $80,000 per life-year.[56]

In response to this problem, the federal government convened a task force on Cost-Effectiveness in Health and Medicine to review issues and questions about the measurement of costs and benefits, the underlying assumptions embedded in cost-effectiveness analyses, and the various perspectives one can assume in conducting cost-effectiveness analyses.[57] The hope was to come up with a recommended standard methodology, but this hope proved to be an elusive goal.

The Ethical Dilemma for Claims of Cost-Effectiveness

Different interests use cost-effectiveness estimates for health promotion interventions for very different purposes.[58] Purchasers and health plans would like to use cost-effectiveness ratios as the basis for assessing the relative value of different health promotion interventions and setting priorities for resource allocation. Providers of health promotion interventions use cost-effectiveness estimates to support their marketing claims about the value of their programs. Advocates for particular interventions also use cost-effectiveness estimates as the basis for arguing for increased resources, much the same way that claims of cost savings are used.[59]

Health promotion advocates argue that their interventions are relatively cost-effective, rather than cost saving, with a much clearer conscience given the scientific evidence available. However, the term "cost-effective" is widely misused and misunderstood. We often hear claims that a health promotion intervention either is or is not cost-effective. But cost-effectiveness is a relative, not an absolute, term. An intervention can only be more or less cost-effective compared with something else.

In addition, many policymakers understand "cost saving" when they hear "cost-effective." Cost-effective does not necessarily mean cost saving. Cost-effective means that the amount of money that must be spent to achieve a desired health outcome is less than the cost of other interventions to achieve the same health outcome. Many more health promotion interventions have been demonstrated to be relatively cost-effective than cost saving, including many immunizations, preventive screenings, and health education programs, but confusion over the meaning of the term cost-effectiveness abounds.

Knowing this, health promotion advocates face another ethical dilemma associated with failing to correct misunderstandings that cost-effectiveness means cost saving. When your audience thinks you mean cost saving, it is equally misleading to argue that health promotion interventions are cost-effective as as it is to claim cost savings in the first place.

What should be done? Do health promotion advocates have an ethical duty to clear up the confusion or, recognizing the political utility of the confusion, continue to perpetuate it?

Conclusion

The story that health promotion advocates need to tell to public and private policymakers is that spending on health promotion and disease prevention can improve the public's health. The efficacy and effectiveness of dozens of health promoting interventions are well established in the scientific literature. There exist only a handful of examples of health promotion interventions that save more in medical care expenditures than they cost to implement.

Policymakers should not look to health promotion interventions as a way to reduce medical care costs. If a healthy population is a goal of our society and maintaining and improving health is valued, then expenditures on health promotion interventions for which there is scientific evidence of effectiveness, measured in terms of improved health as well as relative cost-effectiveness, will move us closer to achieving our goals and demonstrating our values.[60]

The goals of controlling health care costs and promoting the population's health need to be separated and pursued independently. If our goal is to reduce medical care costs, we need to ask how we can reduce costs without harming health. Instead of assuming that HMOs have an incentive to promote the health of their members, we need to ask how we can best hold HMOs accountable for improving the health of their members. Finally, we should not expect to be able to improve health status without incurring some cost. Instead, we need to ask how we can improve health most effectively and efficiently given limited resources.

Health promotion advocates face fundamental ethical dilemmas with respect to their claims for the economic benefits of health promotion. Will they continue to argue that health promotion reduces health care costs (when they know that in most cases it does not), that HMOs promote the health of their enrollees (when they have little incentive to do so), and that health promotion is cost-effective (when many policymakers hear that as cost saving and there are no accepted standards for estimating and comparing cost-effectiveness ratios)? Or will health promotion advocates fight for additional resources to implement health promotion interventions that have demonstrated effectiveness (meaning they improve health) and are relatively cost-effective (meaning that additional resources are needed to improve health status), and hold providers of health promotion interventions accountable for realizing health improvements through contracting?

Continuing to make sweeping generalizations that proclaim the economic medical benefits of health promotion serves no one's interests in the long run and may ultimately produce more harm than good by calling into question the credibility and intellectual integrity of those who care most about promoting and protecting the public's health.

NOTES

1. U.S. Department of Health and Human Services, *An Ounce of Prevention: What Are the Returns?* (Atlanta, Ga: Centers for Disease Control and Prevention, 1993); U.S. Department of Health and Human Services, *For a Healthy Nation: Returns on Investment in Public Health* (Atlanta, Ga: Office of Disease Prevention and Health Promotion and Centers for Disease Control and Prevention, 1994); G. S. Omen, *Prevention: Benefits, Costs, and Savings* (Washington, D.C.: Partnership for Prevention, 1994); J. F. Fries et al., "Reducing Health Care Costs by Reducing the Need and Demand for Medical Care," *NEJM* 329 (1993): 321–25.

2. U.S. Department of Health and Human Services, *An Ounce of Prevention.*

3. U.S. Department of Health and Human Services, *For a Healthy Nation.*

4. Omen, *Prevention: Benefits, Costs, and Savings.*

5. U.S. Department of Health and Human Services, *An Ounce of Prevention.*

6. C. B. Gable, S. S. Holzer, and L. Englehart, "Pneumococcal Vaccine: Efficacy and Associated Cost-savings," *JAMA* 264 (1990): 2910–15.

7. C. C. White, J. P. Koplan, and W. A. Orenstein, "Benefits, Risks and Costs of Immunizations for Measles, Mumps and Rubella," *American Journal of Public Health* 75 (1985): 739–44.

8. Institute of Medicine, *Preventing Low Birthweight* (Washington, D.C.: National Academy Press, 1985).

9. R. M. Scheffler, L. B. Feuchtbaum, and C. S. Phibbs, "Prevention: The Cost-Effectiveness of the California Diabetes and Pregnancy Program," *American Journal of Public Health* 82 (1992): 168–75.

10. J. S. Marks et al., "A Cost-benefit/Cost-effectiveness Analysis of Smoking Cessation for Pregnant Women," *American Journal of Preventive Medicine* 6 (1990): 282–89.

11. U.S. Department of Health and Human Services, *An Ounce of Prevention.*

12. Gable, Holzer, and Englehart, "Pneumococcal Vaccine."

13. White, Koplan, and Orenstein, "Benefits, Risks and Costs of Immunizations."

14. Institute of Medicine, *Preventing Low Birthweight.*

15. Scheffler, Feuchtbaum, and Phibbs, "Prevention."

16. Marks et al., "A Cost-benefit/Cost-effectiveness Analysis."

17. U.S. Department of Health and Human Services, *For a Healthy Nation.*

18. U.S. Department of Health and Human Services, *For a Healthy Nation.*

19. Omen, *Prevention: Benefits, Costs, and Savings.*

20. S. Avruch and A. P. Rackley, "Savings Achieved by Giving WIC Benefits to Women Prenatally," *Public Health Reports* 110, no. 1 (1995): 27–34;

B. Devaney, L. Bilheimer, and J. Schore, "Medicaid Costs and Birth Outcomes: The Effects of Prenatal WIC Participation and the Use of Prenatal Care," *Journal of Policy Analysis and Management* 11, no. 4 (1992): 573–92; P. A. Buescher et al., "Prenatal WIC Participation Can Reduce Low Birthweight and Newborn Medical Costs: A Cost-benefit Analysis of WIC Participation in North Carolina," *Journal of the American Dietetic Association* 93, no. 2 (1993): 163–66; B. Abrams, "Preventing Low Birth Weight: Does WIC Work? A Review of Evaluations of the Special Supplemental Food Program for Women, Infants, and Children," *Annals of the New York Academy of Sciences* 678 (1993): 306–16.

21. Devaney, Bilheimer, and Schore, "Medicaid Costs and Birth Outcomes"; P. A. Buescher et al., "Prenatal WIC Participation."

22. Devaney, Bilheimer, and Schore, "Medicaid Costs and Birth Outcomes."

23. P. A. Buescher et al., "Prenatal WIC Participation."

24. Avruch and Rackley, "Savings Achieved by Giving WIC Benefits to Women Prenatally."

25. R. A. Windsor et al., "Health Education for Pregnant Smokers: Its Behavioral Impact and Cost Benefit," *American Journal of Public Health* 83, no. 2 (1993): 201–06.

26. D. H. Ershoff et al., "Behavioral Health and Cost Outcomes of an HMO-based Prenatal Health Education Program," *Public Health Reports* 98 (1983): 536–47.

27. Ershoff et al., "Behavioral Health and Cost Outcomes."

28. W. J. Hueston, A. G. Mainsou, and J. B. Farrell, "A Cost-benefit Analysis of Smoking Cessation Programs during the First Trimester of Pregnancy for the Prevention of Low-birthweight," *Journal of Family Practice* 9, no. 4 (1994): 353–57.

29. E. E. Bartlett, "Cost-benefit Analysis of Patient Education," *Patient Education and Counseling* 26 (1995): 87–91.

30. C. E. Lewis et al., "Randomized Trial of A.C.T. for Kids," *Pediatrics* 74 (1984): 478–86.

31. Lewis et al., "Randomized Trial of A.C.T. for Kids."

32. W. Neresian, M. Zaremba, and B. Willhoite, "Impact of Diabetes Outpatient Education: Maine," *Morbidity and Morality Weekly Report* 31 (1982): 307–13.

33. Neresian, Zaremba, and Willhoite, "Impact of Diabetes Outpatient Education."

34. D. M. Vickery et al., "Effect of a Self-care Education Program on Medical Visits," *JAMA* 250 (1983): 2952–56.

35. Vickery et al., "Effect of a Self-care Education Program."

36. J. E. Sisk et al., "Cost-effectiveness of Vaccination against Pneumococcal Bacterium among Elderly People," *JAMA* 278, no. 16 (1997): 1333–39.

37. D. M. Huse et al., "Childhood Vaccination against Chickenpox: An Analysis of Benefits and Costs," *Pediatrics* 124, no. 6 (1994): 869–74.

38. K. L. Nichols et al., "The Effectiveness of Vaccination against Influenza in Healthy Working Adults," *NEJM* 333, no. 14 (1995): 889–93; Nichols et al., "The Efficacy and Effectiveness of Vaccination against Influenza among Elderly Persons Living in the Community," *NEJM* 331, no. 12 (1994): 778–84.

39. K. L. Nichols et al., "The Effectiveness of Vaccination against Influenza."

40. K. L. Nichols et al., "The Efficacy and Effectiveness of Vaccination against Influenza among Elderly Persons."

41. R. H. Miller and H. S. Luft, "Managed Care Plan Performance since 1980: A Literature Analysis," *JAMA* 271, no. 19 (1994): 1512–19.

42. Miller and Luft, "Managed Care Plan Performance since 1980."

43. H. H. Schauffler et al., *The State of Health Insurance in California, 1997* (Oakland, Calif.: Regents of the University of California, 1998); H. H. Schauffler and T. Rodriguez, "Availability and Utilization of Health Promotion Programs and Satisfaction with Health Plan," *Medical Care* 32, no. 12 (1994): 1182–96; H. H. Schauffler and S. Chapman, "Health Promotion and Managed Care: Surveys of California's Health Plans and Population," *American Journal of Preventive Medicine* 14, no. 3 (1998): 161–67.

44. Schauffler et al., *The State of Health Insurance in California, 1997;* Schauffler and Chapman, "Health Promotion and Managed Care."

45. Schauffler et al., *The State of Health Insurance in California, 1997.*

46. H. H. Schauffler and T. Rodriguez, "Exercising Purchasing Power for Preventive Care," *Health Affairs* 15, no. 1 (Spring 1996): 73–85.

47. H. H. Schauffler and T. Rodriquez, "Exercising Purchasing Power for Preventive Care."

48. U.S. Department of Health and Human Services, Public Health Service, Agency for Health Care Policy and Research, "Smoking Cessation," *Clinical Practice Guideline No 18,* by M. C. Fiore et al., AHCPR Publication No. 96-0692 (Maryland, April 1996).

49. U.S. Preventive Services Task Force, *Guide to Clinical Preventive Services;* 2nd ed. (Baltimore, Md.: Williams and Wilkins, 1996).

50. U.S. Preventive Services Task Force, *Guide to Clinical Preventive Services;* Institute for Women's Policy Research, *Preventive Health Services: Benefits and Cost-Effectiveness* (Washington, D.C.: Institute for Women's Policy Research, 1994).

51. Centers for Disease Control, "Public Health Focus: Fluoridation of Community Water System," *Morbidity and Mortality Weekly Report* 41 (1992): 372–75, 381.

52. U.S. Department of Health and Human Services, *For a Healthy Nation;* J. Canham-Clyne et al., *Saving Money. Saving Lives: The Documented Benefits of Federal Health and Safety Protections* (Washington, D.C.: Public Citizen Publications, 1995).

53. L. B. Russell, *Educated Guesses: Making Policy About Medical Screening Tests* (Berkeley, Calif.: University of California Press and Milbank Memorial Fund, 1994); Russell, *Is Prevention Better Than Cure?* (Washington, D.C.: Brookings Institution, 1986); K. E. Warner and B. R. Luce, *Cost-Benefit and Cost-Effectiveness Analysis in Health Care: Principles, Practice, and Potential* (Ann Arbor, Mich.: Health Administration Press, 1982); K. A. Phillips and D. R. Holtgrave, "Using Cost-effectiveness/Cost-benefit Analysis to Allocate Health Resources: A Level Playing Field for Prevention? *American Journal of Preventive Medicine* 13, no. 1 (1997): 18–25; M. R. Gold et al., eds., *Cost-Effectiveness in Health and Medicine* (New York: Oxford University Press, 1996); M. C. Weinstein et al., "Recommendations of the Panel on Cost-Effectiveness in Health and Medicine," *JAMA* 276, no. 15 (1996): 1253–58; Institute for Women's Policy Research, *Preventive Health Services*; K. E. Warner and P. A. Warner, "Is an Ounce of Prevention Worth a Pound of Cure? Disease Prevention in Health Care Reform," *Journal of Ambulatory Care Management* 16, no. 4 (1993): 38–49.

54. Gold et al., eds., *Cost-Effectiveness in Health and Medicine*; Weinstein et al., "Recommendations of the Panel on Cost-Effectiveness in Health and Medicine."

55. Warner and Luce, *Cost-Benefit and Cost-Effectiveness Analysis in Health Care*.

56. Warner and Luce, *Cost-Benefit and Cost-Effectiveness Analysis in Health Care*.

57. Warner and Luce, *Cost-Benefit and Cost-Effectiveness Analysis in Health Care*.

58. Warner and Luce, *Cost-Benefit and Cost-Effectiveness Analysis in Health Care*; M. C. Weinstein et al., "Recommendations of the Panel on Cost-Effectiveness in Health and Medicine."

59. Warner and Luce, *Cost-Benefit and Cost-Effectiveness Analysis in Health Care*; Weinstein et al., "Recommendations of the Panel on Cost-Effectiveness in Health and Medicine."

60. H. H. Schauffler et al., "Health Promotion and Disease Prevention in Health Care Reform," *American Journal of Preventive Medicine* 10, no. 5 (supplement) (1994): 1–31.

E. HAAVI MORREIM

Sticks and Carrots and Baseball Bats: Economic and Other Incentives to Modify Health Behavior

In principle, there are many reasons to suppose that, other things being equal, it would be a good thing for people to live healthier lives. After all, adequate health is a precondition for most people to pursue their personal goals and engage in life's rewarding activities. Society is more productive if its citizens are healthy, and limited health care resources can do more good if not wasted on problems that could have been avoided.

Such truisms must not be taken simplistically, however. As noted elsewhere in this volume, it is not always clear which medical interventions and lifestyle changes actually do produce better health or which actually save money.[1] And even if it were definitively known what individuals can effectively do to improve their health, it is one thing to know what is good and another thing to induce people to make major lifestyle changes—and to make them sufficiently long-lasting to produce the desired benefits. Those motivation efforts are the focus of this paper.

Partly because health care is so expensive, and partly because morbidity and mortality are related to conduct,[2] initiatives to modify health-related behavior and to encourage health promotion and disease prevention (HPDP) are becoming widespread. Although health promotion holds some attention, most efforts focus on disease prevention, perhaps because this area is perceived to offer the greatest possibilities for reducing the costs associated with illness and injury. In practical terms, there are three types of prevention: preventable problems, unpreventable problems, and partly preventable problems.

Some illnesses and injuries can, at least in theory, be completely or mostly prevented. Someone who never smokes will not likely die of smoking-related illness; for many people, a long-term, low-fat, high-fiber diet could mean the difference between having and not having significant heart disease or even certain types of cancer; proper immunization can prevent a disease exposure from becoming a disease; and safer sex practices can mean the difference between contracting and not contracting a sexually transmitted disease.

Some illnesses are not preventable but can be detected at a sufficiently early stage to permit medical treatment that can reduce overall morbidity and mortality. Some types of cancer fit this picture.

Chronic illnesses often are neither preventable nor curable. But in many cases acute recurrences, complications, and exacerbations can be avoided or ameliorated. With careful attention to medication and diet, events like asthma attacks, diabetic ketoacidosis, and even some of the long-range complications of diabetes are partly preventable—they can be prevented or at least attenuated.

Each type of prevention requires a rather different sort of behavioral response from the patient. Preventable problems demand attention to one's general lifestyle, including diet, smoking, exercise, avoidance of directly risky behaviors, and adherence to risk-reducing habits such as wearing seat belts and bicycle helmets. Adherence must be high over long periods of time—wearing a helmet on occasion or avoiding cholesterol now and then is essentially useless. Healthy living habits must be the rule and not the exception.

In contrast, early detection of an unpreventable problem typically requires a much more specific behavior: visiting a health care provider's office for periodic screening tests and sometimes for follow-up exams. Here the elements that affect patients' quality of life include whatever costs, discomforts, and embarrassments are associated with the tests themselves, plus ancillary costs and annoyances such as time taken off work or travel expenses.

In further contrast, the chronic illnesses that typify partly preventable problems commonly require a combination of adherence to medications and lifestyle changes considerably more specific and thoroughgoing than those recommended for the general population. The person with heart failure, hypertension, diabetes, arthritis, renal failure, or a variety of other conditions must adhere to a steady regimen of medications, dietary restrictions, and other constraints. The price of even brief failures can be a major episode of illness, long-term aggravation of disability, or even death.

There is overlap among these categories; for example, lifestyle elements figure prominently in both the first and third groups. Still, there are distinct differences in the kinds of behavior required to limit disease at each level. For this reason and because governments, corporations, and health plans all have different tools by which to elicit the desired behavior, it is important to consider the ethical pros and cons of the various incentives that can be levied, which parties do so, and on whom. As the next section will show, there are serious moral limits on the appropriateness of most HPDP incentives.

Who, What, How

Impetus toward HPDP comes mainly from government, from health plans, and from corporate employers.[3]

Government

Public health programs are probably the best-known government-based HPDP initiatives. Because these programs are evaluated elsewhere in this volume,[4] they will not receive substantial attention here. The other major government tools are taxes and laws governing conduct. Taxes on cigarettes and alcohol products, besides collecting in advance some revenue that can be used to cover the health costs incurred by these habits, may also discourage smoking and excessive drinking. Laws regulating conduct include requirements to do certain things, such as to wear helmets or seat belts, or to refrain from things, such as smoking in enclosed public places. While some laws appear under criminal statutes as misdemeanors, others affect the causes of action under civil litigation. Here it is recognized that people are responsible for careless conduct that harms others. Even contributory negligence, such as a failure to comply with recommended medications, can reduce or preclude damage awards for patients who sue their physicians over a bad outcome.[5] And occasionally a patient who knowingly consents to risks, such as an unconventional medical treatment, may simply have to live with a bad outcome, with no right of recovery for injuries.[6]

Arguably, there is at least some room for a government role in HPDP. Public health measures such as sanitation are widely recognized to be crucial to community well-being; reporting requirements for certain transmissible diseases have helped to spare many people from illness; and immunization laws have reduced the prevalence, morbidity, and mortality of several major diseases. Even these are not without some controversy as witnessed, for instance, by debates about whether to require the reporting of HIV infections and, if so, with what protections for confidentiality.

Neither are "sin taxes" uncontroversial. Some observers question the fairness of taxing just a few vices, when we cannot or will not similarly tax things like overeating. One can also observe that many of the people paying these taxes never become ill. Admittedly, it can be replied that those who still create extra risk might reasonably be expected to help pay, even if they never become ill themselves and even if other "guilty" parties go free.[7] As another disadvantage, however, heavy taxes can spawn a black market that may consume as much or more money to catch crooks as it raises for health care.[8] Furthermore, economic facts don't always support the taxes. Smokers do generate health care costs. Yet they often die of relatively inexpensive causes, right around the time of retirement—saving considerably on pension plans.[9] And one recent study actually suggests that nationwide smoking cessation would ultimately raise, not reduce, health care costs.[10]

More fundamentally, government restrictions on citizens' freedom should not be the preferred mechanism for enhancing health. When government says "We forbid you to do X because you might burden the rest of us," it invites major intrusions on human liberty to live as one sees fit. Enforcement could also be highly intrusive, with spying and prying to see who's smoking on the sly. And the invasions can penetrate beyond conduct into private beliefs and values. Health is just one value alongside others ranging from risky sports to admittedly unhealthy ethnic diets. And not everyone agrees what health is.[11] Medical concepts of health and illness are based on scientific notions that can conflict with religious and folk perspectives.[12]

Health Plans

Many health plans are now willing to cover mammography, well-child visits, immunizations, and smoking-cessation programs, and some now offer premium discounts for people who don't smoke or who are willing to enter various HPDP programs.

Other HPDP measures are more specific to managed care. Since prepaid plans do not receive indemnity reimbursement for each service rendered, their incentive ostensibly favors all three sorts of prevention: to help their subscribers avoid illness and injury, to detect disease at an earlier, more treatable (and less costly) stage, and to avoid exacerbations and recurrences of chronic illnesses. Hence, such plans have traditionally covered screenings such as pap smears, annual physical exams, smoking cessation programs, and health education. Even more prominent lately are disease management programs, in which people with chronic illnesses such as asthma are taught in detail about how to keep their symptoms under control.[13]

Despite such an encouraging picture, realities are complex. As a matter of fact, much of HPDP is currently against the economic interests of health plans, however worthwhile it may be for their subscribers. Membership turnover is heavy, and any particular member is likely to be in some other plan within a few years.[14] Because many of the economic and medical rewards of HPDP do not appear for a number of years, it can actually be against a health plan's economic interests to spend large sums of money up front, only to see some other health plan reap the savings.

For preventive interventions oriented toward chronic illness, therefore, it should not be surprising that two of the diseases receiving most prominent attention in disease management programs are asthma and congestive heart failure, for which the savings of averted hospitalizations are immediate rather than distant. Although comprehensive care for diabetes also receives considerable overt attention, in fact many health plans are not entirely faithful in providing recommended tests like annual retinal exams.[15] After all, other than avoiding hospitalizations for diabetic ketoacidosis and certain other acute problems, the rewards of careful diabetes care are not ordinarily garnered until decades after the onset of illness.

The same discordance of incentives likewise hampers many of the interventions oriented toward the first type of prevention, namely avoiding certain problems in the first place. Here, it is not surprising to find a focus on injuries rather than illness, such as encouraging bicycle helmets, in which the savings are foreseeably prompt for each injury prevented.[16] Even here, however, the economic value of such a campaign depends on the particular situation of the party that instituted it. In one case, a hospital reduced bicycle injuries via a helmet campaign and lost $150,000 in reduced emergency room revenues.[17]

This is not to say that health plans only provide HPDP interventions for which they have a direct economic reward. Some are genuinely interested in providing comprehensive and high-quality care. Others are motivated to score well on the HEDIS evaluations to which many corporations look in deciding which health plans to offer their workers.[18] These evaluations include a number of HPDP measures, including frequency of immunizations and mammograms.

Although health plans can offer a variety of HPDP services, they actually have only a limited number of options available for directly enlisting patients' participation. Positive incentives—"carrots"—mainly affect cost-sharing, for instance as a plan might reduce or waive copays, or even present awards to those who participate in wellness programs or reach specified health goals such as weight reduction.

In principle, such positive incentives can be valuable or at least benign. They may or may not inspire major lifestyle change or save enormous amounts of money, but they do set a tone that may help some people enjoy healthier lives. Still, there are challenges. To begin with, it is not clear whether outcomes or efforts should be rewarded.

On the one hand, targeting an outcome may not actually inspire the desired conduct or necessarily inspire the kind of long-term lifestyle changes that could actually make a difference in overall health status. After all, not all people can successfully lose weight because some people are obese for mainly genetic reasons and the temporary losses that go into yo-yo dieting may not be healthy in the long run. An even greater problem for outcomes-oriented incentives may be their inherent tendency to invite gaming of the reward system. In one case, a Minneapolis-based health plan announced a program that would reward people who lost weight. People did lose weight, but not in the way hoped for. Shortly before the deadline, participants purged, starved, took diuretics, and generally did whatever was necessary to get the reward—quite contrary to the program's aspirations of encouraging a general change toward healthy eating and exercise.[19]

Further, it is difficult to determine which outcomes to reward. Should everyone who is close to ideal body weight have a reward? Some health plan members might consider it unfair to reward people simply for having the good fortune to be naturally slender. Yet if the plan rewards only people who have thus far been overweight, then it creates a perverse incentive to engage in the "vice" first and become overweight so that one can qualify for the reward later. Analogously, a plan to reward drug-abusing, pregnant women who quit drugs would in fact reward people for taking up the habit once pregnant, so that their subsequent quitting will qualify for payment.

On the other hand, if effort instead of outcome is the target of the reward system, it can be difficult for health plans to verify who is making the requisite effort—who is truly a nonsmoker, for instance—without intruding unduly on participants' privacy. For instance, some MCOs use their computer information systems to determine which patients receive immunizations and mammograms and who fills and refills their prescriptions.[20] While such monitoring can be helpful as the plan tracks its own inputs and outcomes, it may be somewhat intrusive in the eyes of patients who want to make their own decisions about whether and which tests and medications they wish to take.

Health plans have very limited opportunities to direct negative incentives—"sticks"—toward patients. In principle, they can charge higher premiums and copayments for those with unhealthy lifestyles. But, as noted above, measures for detecting the accuracy of subscribers' reports could intrude seriously on privacy, and simply accepting people's word at face value can reward dishonesty. Further, it is not clear what health plans should do to enrollees who have paid their entire premium but refuse to pay whatever surcharges are imposed after the fact on their undesirable conduct, for instance, when a health plan expects the subscriber to pay extra if his motorcycle accident injuries were worsened by his failure to wear a helmet.[21] Unless the health plan is prepared to spend considerable effort and costs in collection, such extra fees may be more symbolic than real. And again, they may be more likely to inspire gaming behavior than genuine lifestyle change.

A considerably more potent negative tool might be denial of treatment for those whose accident or illness is deemed to be the product of their own behavior. Although health plans have not produced explicit policies of this sort, some physicians have individually expressed willingness to take such measures. Some have refused to offer coronary bypass surgery to patients who refuse to stop smoking,[22] and others would consider denying multiple valve replacements to a patient whose continued intravenous drug use keeps reinfecting his heart.[23]

There are several reasons why this approach must generally be rejected.[24] First, it is not always clear that the behavior is the sole or even primary cause of the health problem. Smoking-related illnesses and obesity, for instance, may be strongly mediated by genetic and environmental factors,[25] and the science behind these putative causal relationships is not always sound. Epidemiologic studies showing links between conduct and health have been overturned on many occasions.[26] Second, the behavior may not be entirely voluntary, as when an addictive component is present. Third, denial of medical care may carry unduly harsh consequences if the person suffers long-term harm or even death simply because he enjoyed the wrong foods or sports. Finally, and this point is perhaps most important, denial of care on grounds of "patient misconduct" can seriously undermine the physician-patient relationship.

Physicians are professionals dedicated to helping people in need, not to executing punitive policies against sinners. Policies denying care to "unworthy" patients must ordinarily be implemented with the aid of the physician who examines the patient and attempts to identify the cause of the problem, in the process of determining what sort of treatment is indicated. Once patients know that their own physicians will be vice-enforcers, they may be much less likely to confide the truths that are often essential to effective care. And when patients are unwilling to trust, the vital physician-patient relationship has been seriously eroded.

The final negative incentive that health plans might levy directly on patients would be nonvoluntary disenrollment from the health plan. This tool, not often used, has been applied mainly for nonpayment of premiums or for fraud. Nevertheless, some health plans are becoming willing to consider removing someone who refuses to do what the plan considers to be his or her part to ensure that health care costs stay within a budget. For self-employed people or those with a preexisting health problem, disenrollment could make it difficult or impossible to find an alternate health plan.

Health plans need not place HPDP incentives directly on patients. They can work indirectly by incentivizing physicians. In these days of economic turbulence and transition, myriad ways of paying physicians open myriad opportunities for fiscal rewards and penalties. Physicians who are paid a capitated fee for all their patients' physician services, for instance, do have an incentive to ensure that people with asthma, congestive heart failure, or other illnesses that can quickly generate large costs are taught to manage their diseases effectively on a day-to-day basis. However, those same physicians have considerably less incentive, if not a counterincentive, to provide preventive care that bears fruit only over the long term.

In other cases, health plans can explicitly award bonuses to physicians who meet specified performance goals for services such as immunizations and mammograms. Here, the goals for the physician can be set to match the goals placed on the health plan itself via the annual HEDIS reviews. As one other tool to incentivize physicians, a health plan can simply deselect from its panel a physician or medical group that does not meet its HPDP goals. It is somewhat like disenrolling patients, although more likely to occur.

In principle, it seems good to encourage physicians to maximize HPDP services for their patients. But these incentives may not always operate benignly. Although some patients will interpret a physician's insistence on screening tests or counseling on lifestyle as a sign of caring, others may regard it as a meddling or nagging that can interfere with their relationship. Reciprocally, many physicians are uncomfortable about the prospect of their patients' perceiving them not as an ally in health but as a parent or vice-cop telling them how to live their lives. These relationship problems are a particular hazard if the patient learns that the physician is being paid a bonus for eliciting specified behaviors from patients.

Even if the patient is unaware of the incentives, such schemes can create a conflict of interest for the physician. Not all patients agree with standard recommendations for, or wish to receive, immunizations and screening tests, for instance. More important, patients with chronic illnesses may not agree to the particular treatment regimen the physician has prescribed. For instance, if the health plan has a very limited drug formulary, a patient's prescribed medications may have side effects that render adherence unacceptable for him. The physician who pressures such a patient into accepting the treatment regimen anyway may dishonor an important principle of medical ethics: the duty to honor each patient's autonomous right to refuse unwanted treatment. Whether the reason is that they don't want side effects, or they disagree with the diagnosis or treatment recommendations, or they have personal priorities other than health care, or they simply don't trust their providers, competent patients have the autonomous right to say "no." Significant financial or other incentives that pressure physicians to pressure patients to comply with HPDP recommendations thus create a potentially problematic conflict.

The intrusion could go further. HPDP often requires patients to make sacrifices—to do things they deem unpleasant (undergo screening tests, take medications with side effects, exercise, wear ugly helmets), or to forgo things they enjoy (favorite foods, smoking, risky avocations). Further, although the sacrifices are ostensibly for the patients' own long-term benefit, others may in fact be the most immediate or even the only beneficiaries. The health plan, not the patient, will save money if it can limit its formulary to cheaper drugs with more side effects, while still inducing patients to take these less desirable medications. Thus, if some particular patient would never have gotten heart disease from his fatty diet, then his sacrifice is essentially for nothing.

The sacrifices may not be solely those of physical comfort. In some instances, faithful adherence to HPDP lifestyles and medical routines can ask the patient to make rather basic changes in personal beliefs. Health-promoting lifestyle changes presuppose that people can actually change the future by things they do today. This view is a personal control-oriented metaphysic that lies at odds with some alternative metaphysical views. Those who are fatalist, for example, whether from religious roots or otherwise, tend to believe that such fundamental matters as the time and manner of one's death or deterioration are in the hands of far greater powers than the lone individual. These people may well view HPDP sacrifices not only as useless, but perhaps even as a kind of hubris, an insult to the powers that be.

Further, those who promote specific HPDP behavior also expect patients to believe that their claims about which actions lead to which outcomes are empirically correct. However, as noted above, epidemiological science has a sometimes notorious history of changing its conclusions. A claim that coffee causes pancreatic cancer is followed by a retraction.[27] Moderate caffeine during pregnancy might—or then again might not—be harmful.[28] Alcohol can be good for your health,[29] and increased dietary fat can diminish your stroke risk,[30] whereas exercise can kill you.[31]

Employers

Corporations have undertaken a variety of HPDP initiatives over the years, including health risk appraisal forms to be filled out by employees (often encouraged via financial incentives to fill them out and in some cases, via further incentives, to share the results with the company); health risk assessments, followed by group and personal counseling on how to enhance health and reduce disease risks; smoking cessation programs (in some cases, forbidding employees to smoke at the work site); special programs for employees with the highest health risks, including high cholesterol, low back pain, diabetes, or arthritis; better cafeteria fare that includes more healthy options and nutritional information; telephone advice and referral services; and employee assistance programs (EAPs) providing counseling for such problems as marital troubles, substance abuse, and stress.[32] Other tactics are more heavy-handed: some firms give overweight workers a choice to lose weight or lose their employer-provided health plan (or pay considerably more for it), while other firms institute random testing for nicotine.[33]

Other measures are not directly applied to employees. A corporation may place direct pressure on its chosen health plans by requiring them to meet certain HPDP goals such as mammography rates, on pain of losing a percent of its premium. Or the company might simply choose among plans on the basis of which has better HPDP programs. Reciprocally, health plans can take the initiative by reducing premiums to companies that are willing to institute designated HPDP measures.[34]

On another level, many corporations opt to self-insure instead of purchasing health plans in the marketplace. Many of these firms contract directly with their own physicians and other providers, either administering the benefits themselves or hiring an outside party to manage such details.[35] These employers can place on physicians various incentives and pressures similar to those created by health plans. Those physicians, in turn, can exert their own influence on patients. In sum, the incentives on patients can be routed in a variety of ways.

Employers can use many of the same tools as health plans to motivate patients and physicians toward HPDP, with basically the same advantages and disadvantages. However, the employer has extra reasons for instituting HPDP measures. Corporations want to save money on health care, of course,[36] but they are also interested in workplace productivity. Ill health, emotional distress, and a variety of other factors can aggravate absenteeism, impede production, and in general reduce efficiency.

To those added reasons, corporations couple an extra tool or two for implementing HPDP. Although a health plan can in principle disenroll a patient for failure to comply with its recommendations, and although the consequences could be severe in certain instances, such tactics are not likely to be used often. Further, if the enrollee can easily enroll in another comparable health plan, the disenrollment may not pose a major problem. In contrast, an employer has the capacity to make compliance with HPDP measures a condition of (continued) employment or job promotion. Some corporations will fire a worker for smoking cigarettes at the work site, for instance, while others may be willing to make salary or wage increases at least partly contingent on meeting company-set health goals. Although it is not known just how widespread such practices are, the possibility of losing one's job or opportunities for advancement may create considerable pressure for an employee to do as the company bids.

A further hazard arises because employers may have greater reason, but less right, than health plans to want access to highly private medical information about their workers, the health plan's patients. The company may be interested in the causes of absenteeism, for instance, or in whether an employee at risk for heart disease is faithfully keeping his cholesterol down. Thus, "A survey of 87 Fortune 500 companies with a total of 3.2 million employees found that 35 percent of respondents used medical records to make decisions about employees. . . . *Consumer Reports* found that 40 percent of insurers disclose personal health information to lenders, employers, or marketers without customer permission."[37] Fears of even the possibility that such information could become known to the employer could prompt workers to be less than truthful with their physicians, or in some instances to avoid health care altogether.

Broader Issues and Avenues for Optimism

In sum, various sticks and carrots can be levied by governments, health plans, and employers, and most of these either focus directly on patients, or indirectly on them through their physicians. As noted above, government's role in HPDP needs to be very limited; health plans should tread carefully lest they invite gamesmanship or, more seriously, imperil the physician-patient relationship or patients' ability to access health care at all; and finally, with their ability to hire, fire, and demote, employers have an even greater potential to make HPDP intrusive rather than helpful.

Throughout these challenges, a more basic issue emerges: identifying the purpose of health care. Initially the question seems too obvious to merit an answer. But the obviousness fades as differences among perspectives emerge. Employers interested in high productivity and low costs, and health plans hoping to contain costs and renew their corporate contracts for another year, might say that health care is intended to make and keep a person as healthy and functional as possible. In contrast, individual people do not necessarily aim to maximize their health in any simplistic way. More often, they may hold rather specific health-related goals, such as to be rid of some particular pain, dysfunction, or illness. Individuals do not always wish to maximize their health overall, given the myriad other priorities that may demand their time, attention, and money. Even if one knows that high-cholesterol foods may shorten one's life, or that a daring sport may cause injury or death, that hazy risk may simply not be as important as the social value of fitting in with one's family and friends, being the object of admiration, or simply carrying on a lifestyle that is familiar and enjoyable.

Another value discrepancy warrants attention. Because corporations and health plans must serve a number of people with a limited budget, their resource goals may especially focus on producing the greatest overall benefit for the total population. Hence, when forced to make choices, they may be more likely to prefer HPDP interventions that could reduce injuries and disease overall, sometimes unavoidably with the downside of providing particular individuals with fewer services than might be optimal. Individuals, in contrast, need to weigh options according to their personal situation. If their care is perceived as free or already paid for, they may want the fastest, most effective, least painful or inconvenient care available, regardless of cost. But if they are paying out of pocket, they may be willing to forgo ideal treatment for the sake of other important projects, whether they be car repairs, tuition, or new clothing.

These competing agendas for health and HPDP need to be juxtaposed against the underlying realities, observed above, that most HPDP requires long-term habits rather than occasional compliance, and that many of the HPDP-promotion methods available to governments, health plans, and employers can invite gaming, intrusiveness, or violations of important relationships. Quite likely, such tactics' odds of successfully creating lifelong lifestyle changes are vanishingly small. Although there may be some room for coercive tactics, particularly where one person's self-destructive conduct imperils other people, it is reasonable to infer that attracting patients' personal agreement with HPDP, rather than trying to impose it or induce transient compliance, is more likely to succeed in the long run and be considerably less morally hazardous.

Some of the best opportunities for such positive attraction may actually come through the workplace. Although employers wield the greatest stick—the threat of firing and demotion—they also hold some of the greatest positive opportunities, since they influence their workers' lives in so many ways. Companies that want to retain their workers over time and minimize costly workforce turnover have a significant interest in those workers' long-term welfare. If a diabetic employee receives good care, both he and the employer can benefit by avoiding or delaying complications such as blindness, amputations, and renal failure. Such considerations currently carry substantial weight, because in a vigorous economy with low unemployment rates, many corporations are concluding that it is more economical to keep their workforce intact than to churn with constant rehiring and retraining. Beyond this, where employers discover that productivity improves when employee morale is high, they may be persuaded that it is best to create positive approaches to health care and HPDP. Many companies have discovered that having and encouraging the use of on-site fitness facilities, for instance, reduces absenteeism, while programs that help patients return to vitality after heart attack or other serious illness can benefit both employer and employee.[38]

If success in HPDP is defined as genuine adherence over long periods of time with minimal gamesmanship, a crucial element of that success may be an emphasis on sociability. Peer approval and social enjoyment can be a far greater motivator than impositions, edicts, or even prize packages. If employers or health plans can create an atmosphere in which HPDP is socially accepted and approved, even enjoyable, then it is more likely that they will see the kind of long-term changes of lifestyle habits that are essential to most HPDP.[39] Thus, an exercise program may be considerably more successful in a context of fun and camaraderie, while weight control may work better in an atmosphere of mutual support and common goals. For firms interested in enticing long-term changes in lifestyle habits, team sports, group fitness activities, cooking classes, and the like may be more attractive options than rigid rules requiring solo reforms. Examples set through active participation by senior management staff may likewise be powerful motivators.

For people with chronic conditions that require medication adherence in addition to lifestyle habits, sociability and mutual support are likewise important. Support groups for people with asthma, diabetes, cancer, and other illnesses can be helpful, not just to boost morale, but to share new ideas and tactics to help one another cope with the adversities of the disease. Beyond this, providers need to exhibit the flexibility that long-term management of a major chronic condition often requires. Unduly restrictive formularies can relegate patients to medications that cause unacceptable side effects and, even if it is otherwise justifiable to limit formularies, it can be medically and economically more efficient to permit exceptions that enhance the patient's ability and willingness to adhere to important regimens. Communication is likewise important. If patients do not feel free to share their concerns, questions, and problems, providers may never have the opportunity to exercise the needed flexibility. Patients need ongoing opportunities to receive answers to their questions, and some health plans have responded by instituting telephone consultation as an adjunct to education classes and physicians' instructions.[40]

If true voluntariness is the key to genuine, sustainable lifestyle improvements of the kind that can actually ward off some illness and injury, it will also be desirable to improve patients' ability to select their health plans, including to switch away from an unsatisfactory plan. At present, 48 percent of employees have only one health plan available;

23 percent have only two plans to choose from; 12 percent have three plans to choose from.[41] Employers can change from one plan to another from one year to the next, often with significant disruptions in physician-patient relationships and thereby in the trust required if physicians are successfully to encourage patients to adopt healthy lifestyles and to manage chronic diseases. Between 1991 and 1993, 41 percent of managed care enrollees who changed plans had to change physicians (compared with only 12 percent of people in fee-for-service plans).[42]

Admittedly, the narrow range of choices so many people now experience and the nonvoluntary switches from one plan to another are largely due to the very real economic constraints that most firms face when determining what benefits to offer their workers. Still, choice of health plan may be crucial to effective HPDP. If patients have the opportunity to choose their own health plans, they are more likely to choose a plan that fits their personal goals and constraints. Perhaps more important, when they have the option to keep or change plans, people can choose to reward a plan that serves them well by staying with it, while penalizing poor service by changing to a different plan. When health plans have the opportunity to retain business by earning patients' loyalty, they are in a much better position to plan for their subscribers' long- and short-range health care. As a consequence, their HPDP initiatives may be better focused, more effective, and more acceptable to patients.

Enhancing choice may not be as difficult as some observers suppose. Many firms are now forming purchasing pools in which they can aggregate their buying power so that they can negotiate better prices for health care and thereby offer a better, wider range of options.[43] In the process, companies have greater opportunity to screen the various health plans from which employees choose. They can require plans to provide HPDP services such as screening exams and nutrition counseling; and as the tools of accountability improve, corporations can also require health plans to demonstrate that their health care efforts actually produce good outcomes. At the same time, health plans competing to be among the available choices and to be reselected by employees can now take much greater interest in that person's long- and short-term health. A major obstacle to serious HPDP—the lack of incentive for health plans to foster enrollees' long-term welfare—is considerably alleviated. An important corollary of such improved patient choice would be risk-rating systems that compensate those health plans enrolling higher numbers of people with chronic illnesses or other high-risk conditions. Only then will it be actually in health plans' interest to win these patients' continued business with high quality of care.[44]

In the final analysis, then, the best tools for effectively bringing patients into HPDP may not be the obvious sticks and carrots and baseball bats. Rather, they may come from the personal inspiration that can emerge only in valued human relationships and from enhancement rather than restriction of choices in health care.

NOTES

1. Helen Halpin Schauffler, "The Credibility of Claims for the Economic Benefits of Health Promotion," *Promoting Healthy Behavior: How Much Freedom? Whose Responsibility?* Daniel Callahan, ed. Georgetown University Press, Washington, D.C., 1999), pp. 37–55.

2. One study concluded that about half of all deaths that occurred in 1990 could be attributed to factors such as tobacco, diet and activity patterns, alcohol and drugs, firearms, sexual behavior, and motor vehicles. See J. M. McGinnis and W. H. Goege, "Actual Causes of Death in the United States," *JAMA* 270 (1993): 2207–12.

3. Several of the arguments in this section are found in an earlier work. See E. Haavi Morreim, "Lifestyles of the Risky and Infamous: From Managed Care to Managed Lives," *Hastings Center Report* 25, no. 5 (1995): 5–12.

3. Beverly Ovrebo, "Health Promotion and Civil Liberties: The Price of Freedoms and the Price of Health," *Promoting Healthy Behavior: How Much Freedom? Whose Responsibility?* ed. Daniel Callahan. (Georgetown University Press, Washington, D.C., 1999), pp. 23–36.

5. B. R. Furrow et al., *Liability and Quality Issues in Health Care* (St. Paul, Minn.: West Publishing, 1991), 188–98.

6. *Schneider v. Revici,* 817 F. 2d 987 (2nd Cir. 1987); *Corlett v. Caserta,* 562 N.E. 2d 257 (Ill. App. 1 Dist. 1990).

7. Robert M. Veatch, "Voluntary Risks to Health: The Ethical Issues," *JAMA* 243 (1980): 50–55.

8. "Canada Mulls Tobacco Tax Cuts to Hit Smugglers," *American Medical News* (7 March 1994), p. 29.

9. W. G. Manning et al., "The Taxes of Sin: Do Smokers and Drinkers Pay Their Way?" *JAMA* 261 (1989): 1604–09.

10. J. J. Barendregt, L. Bonneux, and P. J. van der Maas, "The Health Care Costs of Smoking," *NEJM* 337 (1997): 1052–57.

11. F. Fitzgerald, "The Tyranny of Health," *NEJM* 331 (1994): 196–98.

12. A. Kleinman, L. Eisenber, and B. Good, "Culture, Illness, and Care: Clinical Lessons from Anthropologic and Cross-Cultural Research," *Annals of*

Internal Medicine 88 (1978): 251–88; L. M. Pachter, "Cultural and Clinical Care: Folk Illnesses Benefits and Behaviors and their Implications for Health Care Delivery," *JAMA* 271 (1994): 690–94.

13. H. M. Harris, "Disease Management: New Wine in New Bottles?" *Annals of Internal Medicine* 124 (1996): 838–42; R. S. Epstein and L. M. Sherwood, "From Outcomes Research to Disease Management: A Guide for the Perplexed," *Annals of Internal Medicine* 124 (1996): 832–37; D. K. Greineder, K. C. Loane, and P. Parks, "Reduction in Resource Utilization by an Asthma Outreach Program," *Archives of Pediatric Adolescent* 149 (1995): 415–20; E. R. McFadden Jr. et al., "Protocol Therapy for Acute Asthma: Therapeutic Benefits and Cost Savings," *American Journal of Medicine* 99 (1995): 651–61; K. P. O'Brien, "Managed Care and the Treatment of Asthma," *Journal of Asthma* 32, no. 5 (1995): 325–34; T. V. Hartert et al., "Inadequate Outpatient Medical Therapy for Patients with Asthma Admitted to Two Urban Hospitals," *American Journal of Medicine* 100 (1996): 386–94; M. W. Rich et al., "A Multidisciplinary Intervention to Prevent the Readmission of Elderly Patients with Congestive Heart Failure," *NEJM* 333 (1995): 1190–95.

14. In a 1994 study conducted by the Commonwealth Fund,

> [n]early half of those surveyed reported having changed plans in the past three years. Managed care enrollees were more likely to have done so recently, with 54 percent responding that they had been in their plan for less than three years and only 12 percent for ten years or more, compared with 37 percent of short-term and 26 percent of long-term fee-for-service enrollees. Of those who changes plans, 73 percent reported that the change was involuntary.

See K. Davis et al., "Choice Matters: Enrollees' View of Their Health Plans, *Health Affairs* 14, no. 2 (1995): 99–111, at 103–4.

15. J. P. Weiner et al., "Variation in Office-Based Quality: A Claims-Based Profile of Care Provided to Medicare Patients with Diabetes," *JAMA* 273 (1995): 1503–08; L. L. Leape, "Translating Medical Science into Medical Practice: Do We Need a National Medical Standards Board?" *JAMA* 273 (1995): 1534–37; H. M. Harris, "Disease Management: New Wine in New Bottles?"; R. S. Epstein and L. M. Sherwood, "From Outcomes Research to Disease Management"; L. Page, "Can Plans Manage the Preventive Care Diabetics Need?" *American Medical News* (20 March 1995): 4–5.

16. R. S. Thompson et al., "Primary and Secondary Prevention Services in Clinical Practice: Twenty Years' Experience in Development, Implementation, and Evaluation," *JAMA* 273 (1995): 1130–35.

17. D. M. Berwick, "Quality of Health Care Part 5: Payment by Capitation and the Quality of Care," *NEJM* 335 (1996): 1227–31.

18. D. Borfitz, "Are You Ready for the New Grading System?" *Medical Economics* 72, no. 16 (1995): 151–64; A. Epstein, "Performance Reports on Quality—Prototypes, Problems, and Prospects," *NEJM* 333 (1995): 57–61.

19. "Sinners, Saints, and Health Care: Individual Responsibility for Health" (summary report) (conference sponsored by the Center for Biomedical Ethics of the University of Minnesota, Minneapolis, May 1994), p. 2.

20. R. S. Thompson et al., "Primary and Secondary Prevention Services in Clinical Practice.

21. A. J. Slomski, "Maybe Bigger Isn't Better after All," *Medical Economics* 72, no. 4 (1995): 55–58.

22. M. J. Underwood and J. S. Bailey, "Coronary Bypass Surgery Should Not Be Offered to Smokers," *British Medical Journal* 306 (1993): 1047–48.

23. L. Stell, "The Noncompliant Substance Abuser," *Hastings Center Report* 21, no. 2 (1991): 31–32.

24. For further discussion, see Morreim, "Lifestyles of the Risky and Infamous."

25. W. I. Bennett, "Beyond Overeating," *NEJM* 332 (1995): 673–74.

26. A. R. Feinstein, "Scientific Standards in Epidemiologic Studies of the Menace of Daily Life," *Science* 242 (1988): 1257–63; B. Eskenazi, "Caffeine During Pregnancy: Grounds for Concern?" *JAMA* 270 (1993): 2973–74; G. D. Friedman and A. L. Klatsky, "Is Alcohol Good for Your Health?" *NEJM* 329 (1993): 1882–83: G. D. Curfman, "Is Exercise Beneficial or Hazardous to Your Heart?" *NEJM* 329 (1993): 1730–31.

27. A. R. Feinstein, "Scientific Standards in Epidemiologic Studies of the Menace of Daily Life."

28. Eskenazi, "Caffeine during Pregnancy."

29. Friedman and Klatsky, "Is Alcohol Good for Your Health?"; M. J. Thun et al., "Alcohol Consumption and Mortality among Middle-Aged and Elderly U.S. Adults," *NEJM* 337 (1997): 1705–14.

30. M. W. Gillman et al., "Inverse Association of Dietary Fat with Development of Ischemic Stroke in Men," *JAMA* 278 (1997): 2145–50.

31. Curfman, "Is Exercise Beneficial or Hazardous to Your Heart?"

32. EBRI (Employee Benefit Research Institute). Health Promotion and Disease Prevention: A Look at Demand and Management Programs. Issue Brief number 177 (Sept. 1996); A. J. Slomski, "How Business Is Flattening Health Costs," *Medical Economics* 71, no. 13 (1994): 87–100.

33. G. Jaffee, "Corporate Carrots, Sticks Cut Health Bills," *Wall Street Journal* (3 February 1998), pp. B-1, B-7.

34. Helen Halpin Schauffler and T. Rodriguez, "Exercising Purchasing Power for Preventive Care," *Health Affairs* 15, no. 1 (1996): 73–85.

35. Slomski, "How Business Is Flattening Health Costs."

36. "How Their Bad Habits Can Hurt Your Bottom Line," *Medical Economics* (26 August 1996): 33.

37. L. Sweeny, "Weaving Technology and Policy Together to Maintain Confidentiality," *Journal of Law, Medicine & Ethics* 25 (1997): 98–110.

38. EBRI (Employee Benefit Research Institute), "Health Promotion and Disease Prevention: A Look at Demand Management Programs."

39. Though direct research on the subject is scant, some supportive evidence may come from the literature on physicians and their willingness to change their clinical habits. In recent years' economic upheaval, many physicians have shown a distinct disinclination to change their long-standing habits regarding which tests and treatments they typically order for which illnesses and injuries—even where solid empirical evidence indicates that some of their interventions are unnecessary, and even where education efforts and utilization guidelines urge them to change their patterns. What does seem to work are financial incentives (less gameable here, since the physician's medical orders are openly recorded in patients' charts) together with collegiality and peer pressure from other physicians. See J. Karuza et al., "Enhancing Physician Adoption of Practice Guidelines," *Archives of Internal Medicine* 155 (1995): 625–32; R. L. Lowes, "How Groups Discipline Problem Doctors," *Medical Economics* 72, no. 1 (1995): 45–55; P. B. Ginsburg and J. M. Grossman, "Health System Change: The View from Wall Street," *Health Affairs* 14, no. 4 (1995): 159–63; J. C. Goldsmith, "Driving the Nitroglycerin Truck," *Healthcare Forum Journal* 36, no. 2 (1993): 36–68, 40, 44; D. Blumenthal, "Effects of Market Reforms on Doctors and Their Patients," *Health Affairs* 15, no. 2 (1996): 170–84.

40. J. C. Goldsmith, "Managed Care Comes of Age," *Healthcare Forum Journal* 38, no. 5 (1995): 14–18, 19–20, 22, 24.

41. L. Etheredge, S. B. Jones, and L. Lewin, "What Is Driving Health System Change?" *Health Affairs* 15, no. 4 (1996): 93–104. Obversely, of employers that provide health care, one source indicates that 78 percent offer only one plan, albeit with several products. R. A. Berenson, "Beyond Competition," *Health Affairs* 16, no. 2 (1997): 171–80. Another source indicates that 84 percent provide only one plan. R. J. Blendon, M. Brodie, and J. Benson, "What Should Be Done Now that National Health System Reform Is Dead?" *JAMA* 273 (1995): 243–44.

42. R. A. Berenson, "Beyond Competition."

43. American College of Physicians, "Voluntary Purchasing Pools: A Market Model for Improving Access, Quality, and Cost in Health Care," *Annals of Internal Medicine* 124 (1996): 845–53; Schauffler and Rodriguez, "Exercising Purchasing Power for Preventive Care"; J. C. Robison, "Health Care Purchasing and Market Changes in California," *Health Affairs* 14, no. 4 (1995): 117–30; S. M. Butler and R. E. Moffit, "The FEHBP as a Model for a New Medicare Program," *Health Affairs* 14, no. 4 (1995): 47–61, at 48–51; H. S. Luft, "Modifying Managed Competition to Address Cost and Quality," *Health Affairs* 15, no. 1 (1995): 23–38; T. C. Buchmueller, "Managed Competition in California's Small-Group Insurance Market," *Health Affairs* 16, no. 2 (1997): 218–28.

44. "Without health risk-adjusted payments, health plans and providers have a strong disincentive to compete on quality because they do not want to be known as having the best quality of care for higher-cost illnesses if that would lead to unfavorable selection of enrollees. Without risk-adjusted payments, successful competition based on quality of care could mean substantial financial losses." See R. H. Miller, "Competition in the Health System: Good News and Bad News," *Health Affairs* 15, no. 2 (1996): 107–20, at 168; "Health care delivery systems should not be penalized for attracting and caring for patients with costly chronic conditions. It is irresponsible for purchasers to create powerful incentives for HC systems to avoid caring for sick people. Purchasers should form pools that use risk-adjusted capitation". See A. C. Enthoven, and C. B. Vorhaus, "A Vision of Quality in Health Care Delivery," *Health Affairs* 16, no. 3 (1997): 44–57; see also J. B. Fowles et al., "Taking Health Status into Account When Setting Capitation Rates," *JAMA* 276 (1996): 1316–21; J. P. Newhouse, M. B. Buntin, and J. D. Chapman, "Risk Adjustment and Medicare: Taking a Closer Look," *Health Affairs* 16, no. 5 (1997): 26–43; R. A. Berenson, "Beyond Competition"; A. J. Slomski, "Who Needs HMO's?"

ANN ROBERTSON

Health Promotion and the Common Good: Reflections on the Politics of Need

Ever since Garret Hardin proclaimed the death of the commons in his apocalyptic and highly influential article, "The Tragedy of the Commons," published in *Science* in 1968, the notion of the commons, or the common good, has gone the way of myth.[1] The idea of the common good has persisted, if at all, as a romanticized, idealized, somewhat naive, fairy tale we tell to warm ourselves on blustery winter evenings, which does not really have much to do with the cold, hard, practical realities of social life in the late twentieth century. In the last quarter of this century, public discourse on our common social life has been dominated largely by the classical economic, market view that social life is a matter of autonomous individuals freely contracting with each other to maximize their own individual utility. This radically individualistic view reached its apotheosis with Margaret Thatcher's pronouncement in the early 1980s that "there is no such thing as society, there are only individuals."

This chapter explores the extent to which health promotion offers us a revitalized discourse on the common good. Instead of focusing on ethical issues with*in* health promotion, as my colleagues have so ably done, I would like to consider the possibilities for health promotion to be, in and of itself, an ethical or moral discourse, specifically a discourse on the common good. In making this argument, I am building on the work of others, such as Dorothy Nyswander[2] and Meredith Minkler[3] on the links between health promotion and a social justice agenda, and Dan Beauchamp[4] and Milton Terris[5] on the links between public health and social justice. For the purposes of this chapter, I am assuming a close correspondence between health promotion and public health.

In the last two decades, health promotion and public health have undergone a sea change. The change is a result primarily of efforts to shift health promotion away from the post-Lalonde Report lifestyle behavior focus of the 1970s, and toward a major focus on the social determinants of health—poverty, unemployment, inadequate housing, discrimination, and other social and economic inequities, all of which have significant impacts on the health of people. Underwritten in part by World Health Organization discussion papers,[6] The Ottawa Charter,[7] and initiatives like the Healthy Cities movement,[8] this "new" health promotion places an emphasis on health inequalities, and on the social, political, and economic determinants of those inequalities in health.

This later version of health promotion represented an effort to shift health promotion theory and practice away from individual lifestyle behavior change—like getting people to stop smoking—and toward community development, individual and community empowerment, and healthy public policy. It is this post-Ottawa Charter version of health promotion (the first major document to articulate the principles), with its emphasis on the social determinants of health, that is referred to throughout this chapter. Many would argue that this version of health promotion represents not so much a "new public health" as a return to the historical commitments of public health to social justice.[9]

Most students of health promotion are familiar with the famous 1848 account by Rudolph Virchow of the desperate living conditions of the people of Upper Silesia, which he analyzed as the real causes of their health problems.[10] The great sanitary movement in Britain at the end of the last century was largely driven by health activists, whose efforts at reform were directed at the appalling living and working conditions of the mass of urban poor.[11] As a result of this movement, important public health measures were instituted—"water and sewage were regulated, housing and factory codes were passed, and child labor was prohibited."[12] Attempts throughout the twentieth century to align public health with a social justice agenda reveal the persistence of the moral thrust of public health and health promotion.[13]

My purpose is to consider health promotion as a discourse on the common good and to consider first, the empirical evidence of a connection between health and social justice; second, a possible language of need consistent with health promotion; and third, a particular moral discourse that links health promotion to the pursuit of the common good.

Health and Social Justice

What are the links between health and social justice? To begin with, we have known since the great public health movement of the late nineteenth century that it is the poorest among us who are the sickest, a truth we seem doomed to discover over and over again, even if we wish it to be otherwise. In the late twentieth century, we see this apparently intractable reality in the repeated demonstration of an income gradient for nearly all disease categories—infectious and chronic.

Analyses published in the September 1997 issue of the *American Journal of Public Health* by researchers at the Institute for Social Research at the University of Michigan, on the association between income and all-cause mortality, reinforce this widely observed phenomenon, particularly for people under sixty-five with annual incomes less than $20,000.[14] This research seems to indicate that, up to $20,000 annual income, greater personal wealth does result in greater personal health. Beyond this amount, increased wealth appears to have no additional benefits to health (which may constitute a good prudential argument for a guaranteed minimal income). At this point, there is some debate as to whether the empirical data indicate a gradient or a threshold effect of wealth on health. An additional important finding in this research was the significant negative health effects of persistent income losses for people in the $20,000 to $70,000 per year income bracket, a stark reminder of the very real health effects of job loss and unemployment in an age of "downsizing" and "globalization."

However, the question remains of whether health is a collective (common) good or what exactly the pursuit of health has to do with the pursuit of the common good. I would like to consider briefly two lines of evidence that suggest this link.

The Work of Richard Wilkinson

The first evidence is found in Richard Wilkinson's (1996) most recently published book *Unhealthy Societies: The Afflictions of Inequality.*[15] Wilkinson's comparative analyses of Organization for Economic Cooperation and Development (OECD) data indicate that the effects of wealth on overall health (as measured by national overall life expectancy) is a function *not* of overall wealth (as measured by gross national product), but rather of the size of the wealth gap between the rich and the poor (as measured by Gini coefficients).

Wilkinson's data indicate that those countries with the smaller wealth gap between the richest and poorest had the highest overall life expectancies (for example, The Netherlands and Sweden); the bigger the gap, the lower the overall life expectancy (for example, the United States and Germany). This seems to suggest that inequities in wealth are bad for the health of all of us—rich and poor alike. Granting the limitations of overall life expectancy as a measure of overall health (there are, for example, questions about subgroup rates, about morbidity, and about the desirability of living longer but sicker), nevertheless health indicators such as life expectancy and infant mortality have long been regarded as "canary" measures—that is, indicators that respond quickly and measurably to changes in social and economic conditions.

The Case of Kerala

The second line of evidence linking health and social justice is the case of Kerala. Kerala—a province in southern India—was first analyzed in 1978 by John Ratcliffe, several years before the social determinants of health made their way back into public health.[16] Kerala, one of the poorest provinces in India, had a dismal record in terms of a number of health indicators such as life expectancy, infant and maternal mortality rates, and levels of malnutrition. In the 1950s, a newly elected Marxist provincial government decided not to pursue health goals explicitly, but rather embarked on a broad-based agenda of social and economic improvements, including compulsory education for all children, literacy programs for adults (especially for women), income redistribution, and land reforms to support subsistence agriculture. As a result, a number of health indicators—such as life expectancy, infant mortality, and fertility rates—demonstrated a significant improvement. And the startling thing about this "demographic transition" is that it occurred in the context of Kerala's having levels of income among the lowest in the world. As Ratcliffe observed:

> Indeed, the Kerala experience demonstrates that high levels of social development—evaluated in terms of such quality of life measures as mortality rates and levels of life expectancy, education and literacy, and political participation—*are consequences* of public policies and strategies based not on economic growth considerations but, instead, on equity considerations (emphasis added).[17]

An update of Kerala in 1996 indicated that these broad-based social and economic programs continue to have positive effects on health.[18] The case of Kerala indicates that paying attention to broader issues of equity and social justice has consequences for people's health.

Health and the Common Good

The work of Wilkinson and the case of Kerala suggest that there is something about the way we organize ourselves as a society that has health effects. About his own analyses, Wilkinson says:

> This [strong international relationship between income distribution and national mortality rates] is important for several reasons. First, it appears to be one of the most powerful influences on the health of whole populations in the developed world to have come to light. Second, it seems to be closely related to health inequalities within countries. Beyond that, it has led to an understanding of the significance of the social fabric in developed societies.[19]

This notion is reminiscent of the point that Robert Putnam and others have made recently about "civic society" and "social capital,"[20] such notions that are currently gaining wide popularity.[21] Indeed, it seems, from Wilkinson's data and the case of Kerala, that the pursuit of policies that reduce wealth inequities, and other social/economic policies that redistribute material and nonmaterial resources, has positive *overall* health effects. In other words, the pursuit of health *is* the pursuit of the common good. On the basis of such evidence, I would argue that health promotion—that version of it grounded in the notion of the social determinants of health—represents a moral/ethical enterprise. What health promotion lacks to link it explicitly to the common good is an underlying moral/ethical language.

The Common Good

While a fuller treatment is beyond the scope of this article, it is useful at this point to touch very briefly on what is usually meant by the notion of "the common good," also referred to as the public good, the collective good, the commons, or sometimes by the narrower concept of the public interest. One way of thinking about the common good is that it embraces those things that most people would agree we ought to do and pay for together as benefits of citizenship—things like elementary and secondary education, roads, libraries, clean water, policing, and, in Canada, public broadcasting and Medicare.[22] Economist

John Kenneth Galbraith's concept of public goods included things that cannot be purchased by the individual because they create external benefits for the whole community—things like parks, scientific research, mass transportation, and a clean environment.[23] To others, the common good also refers to intangibles such as commonly held social values, for example, solidarity and justice. What precisely constitutes the common good has long been a philosophical debate, as well as a perennial social and political issue. In other words, "common problems" are common and are characterized primarily by the potential for or actual conflict between individual and collective benefits.

Political scientist Deborah Stone, using the narrower notion of the public interest, says that this notion can have a variety of meanings.[24] One level of meaning could be individual interests held in common, things everybody wants for themselves, such as a high standard of living. Another could be individual goals for the community that may conflict with what individuals want for themselves: a good public education system and low taxes are a case in point. It could also mean goals on which there is some consensus, but this raises questions about whose consensus, what counts as consensus, and the infinitely changing nature of what constitutes the common good. The common good could also mean things that are good for a community qua community, that is, things that ensure the survival of the community, like a minimum of social order and the means of resolving disputes without violence. Stone says that we never have full agreement on the public interest and that "much of politics is people fighting over what the public interest is and trying to realize their own definitions of it."[25]

In "The Needs of Strangers," historian Michael Ignatieff[26] says that a decent and humane society requires a shared language of the good, and that "it is in the language of need that a particular language of the (common) good can be found."[27] Health promotion, by and large, has neglected to deal with the whole need issue at a theoretical or conceptual level. In the next section, I will attempt to articulate a language of need consistent with the notion of health promotion as a discourse on the common good. This takes me to what I have called elsewhere "the politics of need."[28]

The Politics of Need

Ignatieff challenges his readers to find a language of need "adequate to the times we live in,"[29] saying that "modern life has changed the possibilities of civic solidarity, and our language stumbles behind like an overburdened porter with a mountain of old cases."[30] Two of these "old cases" that require unpacking have dominated our discourse on need in the late twentieth century: a therapeutic language of need, and "rights talk."

A Therapeutic Language of Need

Ivan Illich has characterized our age as an age of "disabling professions" in which people had "problems," experts had "solutions," and scientists measured imponderables such as "abilities" and "needs,"[31] as "an age when needs were shaped by professional design."[32] According to John McKnight, this therapeutic approach to need characterizes a service ethic in which citizens are remade as clients or patients, that is, as holders and collections of professionally defined needs.[33] In other words, in the late twentieth century, we have witnessed the commodification of need itself.[34]

This has significant social and political implications, for when people are fragmented into clients of a therapeutic service system, "citizens no longer exist,"[35] the "commons are extinguished,"[36] and politics is indeed in danger of withering away. Robert Bellah and his colleagues argue in their book, *Habits of the Heart,* that the therapeutic mode that pervades both our private and public lives results in the erosion of public and civic life, for "in its quest to reunify the self, the therapeutic attitude distances us from particular social roles, relationships, and practices."[37]

Rights Talk

A second and related language that has dominated our discourse on needs is "rights talk." In her 1991 book, *Rights Talk: The Impoverishment of Political Discourse,* Harvard law professor Mary Ann Glendon critically examines the emergent political discourse in the United States in terms of the "tendency to speak of what is most important to us in terms of rights, and to frame nearly every social controversy as a clash of rights."[38] In policy debates as well as in everyday conversation, claims are made and heard "that whatever right is under discussion at the moment trumps every other consideration."[39]

According to Glendon, American rights talk is characterized by a rhetoric that includes an absoluteness that heightens social conflict and precludes even the possibility of finding common ground; a resounding silence concerning responsibilities—both personal and civic; a neglect of civil society—families, neighborhoods, ethnic and religious associations, and the like—which Glendon believes to be "the principal seedbeds of civic and personal virtue"[40] where "human character, competence, and capacity for citizenship are formed,"[41] and, finally, by an insularity from the moral and political discussions taking place in other western countries with a similar political and philosophical heritage. The key feature of "rights talk" is a "relentless individualism" that conceives of the individual as a lone rights-bearer and, thus, "fosters a climate that is inhospitable to society's losers, and that systematically disadvantages caretakers and dependents, both young and old."[42]

Rights-based language acknowledges only the person who makes a claim against the collective; it rarely considers those against whom the claim is made. In other words, the language of rights says nothing about the responsibility we bear toward one another as members of the community. And finally, as Ignatieff argues, rights-based language is an impoverished language of need:

> Rights language offers a rich vernacular for the claims an individual may make on or against the collectivity. . . . It is relatively impoverished as a means of expressing individuals' needs *for* the collectivity.[43]

In responding to Ignatieff's challenge for a new language of need, I suggest that a renewed language of need is one that links need with the life of the community.

Needs and the Life of the Community

It could be said that the recognition of the existence of fundamental human needs represents the underlying catalyst for the formation of all human communities. Hegel characterized civil society as a "system of needs."[44] And Stone says "much of politics is . . . an effort to define need collectively."[45] Indeed, it could be argued that the primary purpose of politics is the definition and discussion of issues of human needs, for "the social contract is an agreement to reach decisions together about what goods are necessary to our common life, and then to provide those goods for one another."[46]

It could be argued that any group or community is essentially characterized by the kinds of needs it collectively provides for, and the extent to which it provides for those needs. Those needs that a society or community decides are necessary to the common life, Stone calls "public needs," about which she says: "The pattern of public needs is the signature of a society. In its definition of public needs, a society says what it means to be human and to have dignity in that culture."[47]

Stone considers that "communal provision . . . may be the most important force holding communities together."[48] As political scientist Michael Walzer puts it, "Political community for the sake of provision, provision for the sake of community: the process works both ways and that is perhaps its crucial feature."[49]

In a similar spirit, and in opposition to the prevailing economic view of human behavior,[50] Ignatieff says:

> It is as common for us to need things on behalf of others, to need good schools for the sake of our children, safe streets for the sake of our neighbours, decent old people's homes for the strangers at our door, as it is for us to need them for ourselves. *The deepest motivational springs of political involvement are to be located in this human capacity to feel needs for others* (emphasis added).[51]

Walzer argues that it is through the collective provision of public needs that the community recognizes membership in the community. In addition, the extent of and inclusiveness in the discussion about need in any particular community is significant, for "when all the members share in the business of interpreting the social contract, the result will be a more or less *extensive system of communal proviso*" (emphasis added).[52]

Post-Ottawa Charter health promotion, with its emphasis on the broad social determinants of health is, like public health, fundamentally about community, about the shared values of life, health, and security, and is, thus, in and of itself, a discourse on the common good.[53]

Health Promotion and the Pursuit of the Common Good

"[I]ndividual freedom and the general welfare alike depend on the condition of the fine texture of civil society—on a fragile ecology for which we have no name."[54]

I suggest that the "fragile ecology for which we have no name" be named a "moral economy of interdependence." I offer a moral economy of interdependence as a particular language of need appropriate to a health promotion based on the broad social determinants of health. I conclude with an exploration of what a moral economy of interdependence might look like, and how it might speak to health promotion as a discourse on the common good. My first task is to explicate the notions of "moral economy" and "interdependence."

Moral Economy: The Notion of Reciprocity

The moral issue at the heart of any society is this: When does need entitle people to make a claim against the collective? Any given society's answer to this question is embodied in what has been called the "moral economy." Moral economy has been defined as "the collectively shared basic moral assumptions constituting a system of reciprocal relations"[55]— that is, it is about our "collectively shared assumptions defining norms of reciprocity."[56] Deborah Stone characterizes the concept of moral economy thus:

> The moral economy of a society is its set of beliefs about what constitutes just exchange: not only about how economic exchange is to be conducted in normal times but also, . . . when poor individuals are entitled to social aid, when better-off people are obligated to provide aid, and what kinds of claims anyone—landowners, employer, governments—can legitimately make on the surplus product of anyone else.[57]

In his book, *The Gift Relationship,* Richard Titmuss,[58] that passionate defender of the underlying moral principles of the modern welfare state, uses the case of voluntary blood donation to provide an eloquent articulation of what shared moral economy assumptions of reciprocity might look like:

> In not asking for or expecting any payment of money, these donors signified their belief in the willingness of other men to act altruistically in the future, and to combine together to make a gift freely available should they have a need for it. *By expressing confidence in the behaviour of future unknown strangers they were thus denying the Hobbesian thesis that men are devoid of any distinctively moral sense* (emphasis added).[59]

This description is in marked contrast to market-based notions of reciprocity. The emerging concept of "social capital," referred to earlier, also invokes moral economy notions of reciprocity. Social capital "refers to features of social organization, such as networks, norms, and trust, that facilitate coordination and cooperation for mutual benefit."[60] The important thing about social capital is that it is a public good and that, unlike physical capital, it increases with use. As Putnam says, "a society that relies on generalized reciprocity is more efficient than a distrustful one."[61]

Also, in contrast to what Bellah et al. call a "giving/getting" notion of reciprocity,[62] or to more narrowly based discussions of rights and entitlements, the concept of moral economy is as much about our obligations to one another as it is about the claims we are entitled to make against each other. In other words, the language of moral economy acknowledges both sides of the reciprocity equation. Clearly, this way of thinking about reciprocity differs significantly from liberal or market-place notions of reciprocity, for it acknowledges our fundamental inter-dependence.

Interdependence: Beyond the Dependence/Independence Dichotomy

The issue of "dependency" underlies the majority of social policy debate in the modern welfare state. Most social policy is made on the basis that to be "dependent" is bad and to be "independent" is good. One of the more significant legacies from the European Enlightenment—in terms of its social and political implications—which informs most contemporary liberal debate, is a radical individualism in which the individual is regarded both as a "lone rights bearer"[63] and as an autono-mous moral agent.[64] Deriving from Locke's and Rousseau's notion of "natural man" as a solitary self-sufficient creature and Kant's notion of man as a freely choosing, rational actor,[65] this kind of individualism pays "extraordinary homage to independence and self-sufficiency, based on an image of the rights-bearer as a self-determining, unencumbered individual, a being connected to others only by choice."[66]

However, for all the symbolic power of the rhetoric of independence, as Glendon wryly observes, this mythic lone individual "possesses little resemblance to any living man, and even less to most women."[67] The concept of interdependence, on the other hand, embraces the notion that our good or bad fortune, our achievements or failures are never entirely "ours." In his book, *Liberalism and the Limits of Justice,* Mark Sandel writes of our indebtedness—and, therefore, reciprocal obligation—to others in the larger context within which we live.

> [I]t seems reasonable to suppose that what at first glance appears as "my" assets are more properly described as common assets in some sense; since others made me, and in various ways continue to make me, the person I am, it seems appropriate to regard them, in so far as I can identify them, as participants in "my" achievements and common beneficiaries of the rewards they bring. . . . [Thus] we may come to regard ourselves . . . as participants in a common identity, be it a family or community or class or people or nation.[68]

In other words, the fact that we live in communities means that we are ispo facto interdependent. By transcending the dependence/independence dichotomy with the concept of interdependence, we cut to the essence of human need in the context of the community. The modern welfare state, whose rapid, near global demise we are currently witnessing, represents an administrative attempt to extend this concept of interdependence to those whom Ignatieff calls "the strangers at my door,"[69] a perspective that I have addressed elsewhere.[70]

Toward a Moral Economy of Interdependence

I have responded to Ignatieff's challenge to come up with a language of need that can speak to the times in which we live with the concept of a "moral economy of interdependence." A moral economy of interdependence acknowledges that we are always already embedded in webs of mutual dependence and that, therefore, the pursuit of the common good is always, already contiguous with the pursuit of our own individual good. Indeed, our very individuality is social, created, sustained, ensured, and protected by the community,[71] for "humanity is the gift of society to the individual."[72] I conclude with a brief discussion of what a moral economy of interdependence—as an alternative language of need—might look like.

First of all, we must readmit the language of moral reasoning into discussions of public health policy and practice. Moral and political language has been replaced, in part, by therapeutic language. Because the therapeutic self defines situations in terms of its own wishes and wants, the question is not "Is this right or wrong?" but rather "Does this work for me?"

> In asserting a radical pluralism and the uniqueness of each individual, [the therapeutically inclined] conclude that there is no moral common ground and therefore no public relevance of morality outside the sphere of minimal procedural rules and obligations not to injure.[73]

The result of this kind of thinking is a kind of moral relativism, or perhaps more accurately a kind of moral nihilism. It is difficult to imagine how any notion of community—or, indeed, vision for public health—can be built on the basis of a therapeutic language.

Recent attempts by philosophers, communitarians, feminists, and others to revitalize political discourse with moral reasoning all dismiss the liberal notion of the individual as an autonomous moral agent, and seek to place the individual back into the moral context of the community.[74] The question from this place becomes "What kind of community or society do we want to live in?" In his book, *After Virtue,* philosopher

Alasdair MacIntyre argues for such a social morality, saying that "the only grounds for the authority of laws and virtues can only be discovered by entering into those relationships which constitute communities whose central bond is a shared vision of and understanding of goods."[75] This is related to, but not identical with, the notion of social capital, discussed earlier, which is created through civic engagement and which has been referred to as a "moral resource."[76]

A moral economy of interdependence would also seek to decommodify the notion of reciprocity, by recognizing that not all human exchanges can be entered into a cost-benefit analysis. Examples include love, time, energy, kindness, commitment, shared memories, care— all things that constellate human relationships and create community. The relative absence of these kinds of considerations in most public health policy discussions has significant implications for issues of equity and social justice. As Alan Walker says, speaking specifically of the care of the elderly:

> Since the commodified form of social relations implicit in neo-classical economics undervalues both the role of older people and the unpaid work of carers (more important in the life worlds of older people than formal care), there is an antagonistic relationship between the needs of older people and their families and the assumptions underlying macroeconomic policy. In other words, raw neo-classical macroeconomics is unlikely to produce an equitable outcome in resource distribution for older people (or anyone else for that matter).[77]

A moral economy of interdependence would not only take need out of the marketplace where it is commodified, it would also take it out of the courts where needs are reconceptualized as rights. Arguing that "our rights-laden public discourse easily accommodates the economic, the immediate, and the personal dimensions of a problem, while it regularly neglects the moral, the long-term, and the social implications,"[78] Glendon advocates for balancing the rhetoric of rights with the language of responsibility and reciprocity. It is for this reason that many contemporary social policy analysts[79] argue for a repoliticization of need by placing the discussion and arbitration of issues of need back into the *polis.*[80]

To repoliticize need would mean to curb the power of the "experts" and the growth of the "therapeutic state," and involve people and communities in determining their own needs and the most appropriate ways to meet them. Educators, community organizers, and public health activists like Paolo Freire,[81] Saul Alinsky,[82] John McKnight,[83] and Meredith Minkler[84] demonstrate ways in which this can be accomplished. Health promotion concepts such as "empowerment"[85] and "community development,"[86] and public health initiatives like "Healthy Cities"[87] represent efforts to repoliticize need within the health domain.

Others have invoked this principle of interdependence in relation to public health. In arguing for an ecological base for public health, Kickbusch says that "interdependence is central to ecological thinking."[88] In ecological terms, health is seen as "a fundamental resource to the individual, the community and to society."[89] Doyal and Gough argue further that "the protection of the health of individuals, their learning and the growth of their emotional maturity are themselves social processes."[90] The pursuit of health, thus, *is* the pursuit of the common good. And health promotion, as a moral enterprise, stands as one discourse on the common good.

Conclusion

A fundamental conviction of this chapter is that words and ideas matter. It matters that we speak a language of need in terms of moral economy and interdependence, rather than in terms of moral nihilism and radical individualism. Words matter because "what we cannot imagine and express in language has little chance of becoming a sociological reality,"[91] for "the way we name things and discuss them shapes our feelings, judgments, choices, and actions, including political actions."[92]

Likewise, ideas matter because "the essence of policy making in political communities [is] the struggle over ideas. Ideas are a medium of exchange and a mode of influence even more powerful than money and votes and guns. Shared meanings motivate people to action and meld individual striving into collective action."[93]

Examining our ideas matters because "our strongest bulwark against demagoguery is the habit of critical discussion about and self-conscious awareness of the public ideas that envelop us."[94] The public ideas and language that currently envelop us are those of the market, corporatism, fiscal constraint, and globalization—ideas that are driving the nearly universal dismantling of the welfare state and eroding any notion we might have of the common good. Health promotion offers us the possibility of a countervailing discourse.

From its beginning, health promotion has been fundamentally a moral enterprise, orienting its efforts toward improving the life chances of the most disadvantaged of society's members. There is an increasing body of evidence that it is wealth and social inequalities that create health inequalities.[95] But as one writer so eloquently puts it: "the growing gap between rich and poor has not been ordained by extraterrestrial beings. It has been created by the policies of governments."[96] It is health promotion, in part through rediscovery and articulation of its moral underpinnings in the language of a moral economy of interdependence, that offers us a renewed public discourse on the common good.

NOTES

1. Garret Hardin, "The Tragedy of the Commons," *Science* 162 (1968): 1243–48.

2. Dorothy Nyswander, "The Open Society: Its Implications for Health Educators," *Health Education Monographs* 1 (1967): 3–13.

3. Meredith Minkler, "Health Education, Health Promotion and the Open Society: An Historical Perspective," *Health Education Quarterly* 16, no. 1 (1989): 17–30.

4. Dan E. Beauchamp, "Public Health as Social Justice," *Inquiry* 12, no. 1 (1976): 3–14.

5. Milton Terris, "Determinants of Health," *Journal of Public Health Policy* 14, no. 2 (1994): 5–17.

6. See, for example, World Health Organization, "Health Promotion: A Discussion Document on the Concepts and Principles," *Health Promotion* 1, no. 1 (1986): 73–76.

7. Government of Canada, "Ottawa Charter for Health Promotion," *Health Promotion* 1, no. 4 (1986): iii–v.

8. J. Ashton, *Healthy Cities* (Bristol, U.K.: Open University Press, 1993); Len Duhl, "The Healthy City: Its Function and Its Future," *Health Promotion* 1, no. 2 (1986): 55–60.

9. Ilona Kickbusch, "Approaches to an Ecological Base for Public Health," *Health Promotion* 4, no. 4 (1989): 265–68; Ron Labonte, *Health Promotion and Empowerment: Practice Frameworks* (Toronto: Centre for Health Promotion/Participation, 1993); Simon Szreter, "The Importance of Social Intervention in Britain's Mortality Decline c. 1850–1914: A Re-interpretation of the Role of Public Health," *Society for the Social History of Medicine* 1, no. 1 (1988): 1–41.

10. Sylvia Tesh, *Hidden Arguments: Political Ideology and Disease Prevention Policy* (New Brunswick and London: Rutgers University Press, 1990).

11. Simon Szreter, "The Importance of Social Intervention."

12. Avi Y. Ellencweig and Ruthellen B. Yoshpe, "Definition of Public Health," *Public Health Review* 12 (1984): 65–78.

13. See, for example, Beauchamp, "Public Health as Social Justice"; Kickbusch, "Approaches to an Ecological Base for Public Health"; Labonte, *Health Promotion and Empowerment: Practice Frameworks*; Minkler, "Health Education,

Health Promotion and the Open Society: An Historical Perspective"; Nyswander, "The Open Society: Its Implications for Health Educators"; Terris, "Determinants of Health."

14. Peggy McDonough et al., "Income Dynamics and Adult Mortality in the United States, 1972 through 1989," *American Journal of Public Health* 87, no. 9 (1997): 1476–83.

15. Richard G. Wilkinson, *Unhealthy Societies: The Affliction of Inequality* (London: Routledge, 1996).

16. John Ratcliffe, "Social Justice and the Demographic Transition: Lessons from India's Kerala State," *International Journal of Health Services* 8, no. 1 (1978): 123–44.

17. Ratcliffe, "Social Justice and the Demographic Transition," p. 140.

18. Bill McKibben, "The Enigma of Kerala," *Utne Reader* (March–April 1996): 103–12.

19. Wilkinson, *Unhealthy Societies,* p. 4.

20. See, for example, Robert D. Putnam, "The Prosperous Community: Social Capital and Public Life," *American Prospect* 13 (Spring 1993): 35–43; Putnam, *Making Democracy Work* (Princeton, NJ: Princeton University Press, 1993); Putnam, "Bowling Alone: America's Declining Social Capital," *Journal of Democracy* 6, no. 1 (1995): 65–78; Putnam, "The Strange Disappearance of Civic America," *American Prospect* 24 (Winter 1996): 34–48.

21. While a fuller discussion of the diverse interpretations (theoretical and political) and applications (at the micro-, meso-, or macrolevel of social organization) of the notion of "social capital" or, as it is sometimes called, "social cohesion" is beyond the scope of this chapter, it is important to note here that this concept has been explicitly linked to health. See, for example, Ichiro Kawachi et al., "Long Live Community: Social Capital as Public Health," *American Prospect* 35 (November–December 1997): 56–59. Wilkinson is clearly making this point in the selection quoted.

22. Canadian Broadcasting Corporation, *The Public Good Reader* (Toronto: Author, 1996), p. 1.

23. Canadian Broadcasting Corporation, *The Public Good Reader,* p. 4.

24. Deborah A. Stone, *Policy Paradox and Political Reason* (Glenview, Ill.: Scott Foresman/Little Brown College Division, 1988).

25. Stone, *Policy Paradox and Political Reason,* p. 15.

26. Michael Ignatieff, *The Needs of Strangers* (Harmonsworth, UK: Penguin Books, 1984).

27. Ignatieff, *The Needs of Strangers,* p. 14.

28. Ann Robertson, "Critical Reflections on the Politics of Need: Implications for Public Health," *Social Science and Medicine* (forthcoming).

29. Ignatieff, *The Needs of Strangers,* p. 141.

30. Ignatieff, *The Needs of Strangers,* p. 138.

31. Ivan Illich, "Disabling Professions," in *Disabling Professions,* ed. Ivan Illich et al. (London: Marion Boyars, 1977), p. 11.

32. Illich, "Disabling Professions," p. 13.

33. John McKnight, "Professionalized Service and Disabling Help," in *Disabling Professions,* ed. Ivan Illich et al. (London: Marion Boyars, 1977).

34. See Dan E. Beauchamp, *The Health of the Republic: Epidemics, Medicine, and Moralism as Challenges to Democracy* (Philadelphia: Temple University Press, 1988) for a discussion of this issue as it relates to public health.

35. McKnight, "Professionalized Service and Disabling Help," p. 85.

36. Illich, "Disabling Professions," p. 27.

37. Robert Bellah et al., *Habits of the Heart: Individualism and Commitment in American Life* (New York: Harper & Row, 1985), p. 127.

38. Mary Ann Glendon, *Rights Talk: The Impoverishment of Political Discourse* (New York: The Free Press, 1991), p. 4.

39. Glendon, *Rights Talk,* p. 8.

40. Glendon, *Rights Talk,* p. 14.

41. Glendon, *Rights Talk,* p. 109.

42. Glendon, *Rights Talk,* p. 14.

43. Ignatieff, *The Needs of Strangers,* p. 113.

44. Patricia Springborg, *The Problem of Human Needs and the Critique of Civilization* (London: George Allen & Unwin, 1981).

45. Stone, *Policy Paradox and Political Reason,* p. 81.

46. Michael Walzer, *Spheres of Justice* (New York: Basic Books, 1983), p. 65.

47. Stone, *Policy Paradox and Political Reason,* p. 81.

48. Stone, *Policy Paradox and Political Reason,* p. 82.

49. Walzer, *Spheres of Justice,* p. 64.

50. However, for a recent challenge to the neoclassical economics view of "economic man" as a rational actor who makes individual rational choices in the marketplace of goods and services on the basis of endogenous preferences, see Robin Hahnel and Michael Albert, *A Quiet Revolution in Welfare Economics* (Princeton, NJ: Princeton University Press, 1990).

51. Ignatieff, *The Needs of Strangers,* p. 17.

52. Walzer, *Spheres of Justice,* p. 83.

53. Beauchamp, "Public Health as Social Justice"; Ignatieff, *The Needs of Strangers.*

54. Glendon, *Rights Talk,* pp. 109–10.

55. Martin Kohli, "Retirement and the Moral Economy: An Historical Interpretation of the German Case," in *Critical Perspectives on Aging: The Political and Moral Economy of Growing Old,* ed. Meredith Minkler and Carroll L. Estes (Amityville, NY: Baywood Publishing, 1991), p. 275.

56. Meredith Minkler and Tom Cole, "Political and Moral Economy: Not Such Strange Bedfellows," in *Critical Perspectives on Aging: The Political and Moral Economy of Growing Old,* ed. Meredith Minkler and Carroll L. Estes (Amityville, NY: Baywood Publishing, 1991), p. 38.

57. Stone, *Policy Paradox and Political Reason,* p. 19.

58. Richard M. Titmuss, *The Gift Relationship* (Harmonsworth, UK: Penguin Books, 1973).

59. Titmuss, *The Gift Relationship,* p. 269.

60. Putnam, "The Prosperous Community: Social Capital and Public Life," pp. 35–36.

61. Putnam, "The Prosperous Community: Social Capital and Public Life," p. 37.

62. Bellah et al., *Habits of the Heart.*

63. Glendon, *Rights Talk.*

64. Alasdair MacIntyre, *After Virtue: A Study in Moral Theory* (Notre Dame, Ind.: University of Notre Dame Press, 1984); Michael J. Sandel, *Liberalism and the Limits of Justice* (Cambridge: Cambridge University Press, 1982).

65. Springborg, *The Problem of Human Needs and the Critique of Civilization.*

66. Glendon, *Rights Talk,* p. 48.

67. Glendon, *Rights Talk,* p. 48.

68. Sandel, *Liberalism and the Limits of Justice,* p. 143.

69. Ignatieff, *The Needs of Strangers,* p. 16.

70. Robertson, "Critical Reflections of the Politics of Need: Implications for Public Health."

71. Bellah et al., *Habits of the Heart.*

72. Len Doyal and Ian Gough, *A Theory of Human Need* (London: MacMillan, 1991), p. 78.

73. Bellah et al., *Habits of the Heart,* p. 141.

74. See, for example, Bellah et al., *Habits of the Heart;* Bellah et al., *The Good Society* (New York: Alfred A. Knopf, 1991); Nancy Fraser, "Talking about Needs: Interpretive Contests as Political Conflicts in Welfare-state Societies," in *Feminism & Political Theory,* ed. Cass R. Sunstein (Chicago and London: University of Chicago Press, 1990); Elizabeth Frazer and Nicola Lacey, *The Politics of Community: A Feminist Critique of the Liberal-Communitarian Debate* (Toronto: University of Toronto Press, 1993); Marilyn Friedman, "Beyond Care: The De-Moralization of Gender," in *An Ethic of Care: Feminist and Interdisciplinary Perspectives,* ed. M. J. Larrabee (New York and London: Routledge, 1993); Glendon, *Rights Talk;* Ignatieff, *The Needs of Strangers;* MacIntyre, *After Virtue;* Sandel, *Liberalism and the Limits of Justice;* Joan C. Tronto, *Moral Boundaries: A Political Argument for an Ethic of Care* (New York and London: Routledge, 1993).

75. MacIntyre, *After Virtue,* p. 258.

76. Putnam, "The Prosperous Community: Social Capital and Public Life," *American Prospect* 13, (Spring 1993): 35–43, at 37.

77. Alan Walker, "The Economic 'Burden' of Ageing and the Prospect of Intergenerational Conflict," *Ageing and Society* 10 (1990): 377–96, at 385.

78. Glendon, *Rights Talk,* p. 171.

79. For example, Bellah et al., *The Good Society;* Glendon, *Rights Talk;* Ignatieff, *The Needs of Strangers;* Robert B. Reich, *The Power of Public Ideas*

(Cambridge, Mass.: Ballinger Publishing, 1988); Stone, *Policy Paradox and Political Reason.*

80. *Polis* is used here, similar to its classical Greek usage (Stone, *Policy Paradox and Political Reason*), to refer to the entire domain of public discourse, and not just the more narrow sense of "political" in terms of the institutionalized official governmental system. According to Nancy Fraser, "something is 'political' if it is contested across a range of different discursive arenas and among a range of different publics." See Fraser, "Talking about Needs," p. 165.

81. Paulo Freire, *Pedagogy of the Oppressed* (New York: Continuum, 1988).

82. Sol Alinsky, *Rules for Radicals* (New York: Random House, 1972).

83. McKnight, "Regenerating Community," *Social Policy* (Winter 1987): 54–58.

84. Meredith Minkler, "Improving Health through Community Organization," in *Health Behavior and Health Education: Theory, Research and Practice* ed. K. Glanz et al. (Oxford: Jossey-Bass, 1990).

85. Labonte, *Health Promotion and Empowerment: Practice Frameworks;* Nina Wallerstein, "Powerlessness, Empowerment and Health: Implications for Health Promotion Programs," *American Journal of Health Promotion* 6, no. 3 (1992): 197–205.

86. A. Beattie, "Community Development for Health: From Theory to Practice," *Radical Health Promotion* 4 (1986): 12–18; Wendy Farrant, *"Health for All" in the Inner City: Proposed Framework for a Community Development Approach to Health Promotion Policy and Planning at a District Level* (London: Paddington and North Kensington Health Authority, 1986); J. Lotz, "Community Development: A Short History," *Journal of Community Development,* (May–June 1987): 41–46.

87. Ashton, *Healthy Cities*; Duhl, "The Healthy City."

88. Ilona Kickbusch, "Approaches to an Ecological Base for Public Health," *Health Promotion* 4, no. 4 (1989): 265–68, at 265.

89. Kickbusch, "Approaches to an Ecological Base," p. 267.

90. Doyal and Gough, *A Theory of Human Need,* p. 79.

91. Bellah et al., *Habits of the Heart,* p. 15.

92. Glendon, *Rights Talk,* p. 11.

93. Stone, *Policy Paradox and Political Reason,* p. 7.

94. Reich, *The Power of Public Ideas,* p. 10.

95. See the entire issue of the *British Medical Journal* 312 (April 20, 1996) for an in-depth discussion of this topic.

96. Peter Montague, "Economic Inequality and Health," *Rachel's Environment & Health Weekly* 497 (June 6, 1996).

RONALD LABONTE

Health Promotion
and the Common Good:
Toward a Politics of Practice

One of the ethical dilemmas facing health promotion/disease prevention (HP/DP) work is to find a balance between respect for personal rights and interventions for the common good that may restrict individual liberty. This dilemma corresponds to two broadly divergent theories of the common good: Libertarian or neoliberalism and its emphasis on individual autonomy, and social justice or communitarianism and its emphasis on the collectivity. Libertarians hold that individual autonomy is the superordinate human goal and that the rational pursuit of self-interest, particularly economic self-interest, is ultimately utilitarian, creating the greatest good for the greatest number.[1] The political problem becomes one of ensuring personal freedom against interferences from the collective in the form of state regulation, except in very limited circumstances. Social justice adherents argue that individual responsibilities to others is the superordinate human goal and certain forms of private behaviors, particularly economic or market activities, must be collectively regulated.[2] The political problem becomes one of using state or community norms to ensure that utilitarian goals are socially just.

In this chapter I argue against a libertarian theory for the common good in favor of a social justice theory. I illustrate my argument by reference to two recent attempts in Canada to formulate ethical principles for health promotion practice. The first was a "stock-taking" exercise on health promotion practice that involved over one thousand practitioners and academics and culminated in the consensus document, *Action Statement on Health Promotion in Canada.*[3] The second was a two-year critical reflection project involving over fifty staff at the Toronto public health department, considered one of the international "innovators" in health promotion practice.[4]

Libertarianism's Contribution: Respect for Autonomy

Libertarianism's emphasis on individual autonomy forms one of the "*prima facie* principles" in health care ethics.[5] This deontological, or rights-oriented, ethic challenges the practice of unequal power relations between health professionals and patients/clients. Some of this inequality may be unavoidable. The professional may have more information on a person's disease or treatment options, or may occupy a gatekeeping role to other services. But some of this inequality may be coercive, such as the assumption that professional knowledge is fact while client knowledge is opinion, or the discursive means by which professionals seek to obtain compliance.[6] In HP/DP, this problem is taken up in the idea of empowerment[7] and its implicit or explicit critiques of professionalism as a system of dominance.[8] This empowerment concern was expressed in the first principle in the *Action Statement*: Individuals are treated with dignity and their innate self-worth, intelligence, and capacity of choice are respected.

This emphasis on capacity of choice arose from criticisms that HP/DP commonly assumes that unhealthy individual behaviors are irrational (unintelligent) or irresponsible. Early critics of the "victim blaming" potential of a behavioral approach also gave short shrift to the issue of individual autonomy, or capacity of choice, arguing that such "structural" health determinants as poverty or racism represented conditions over which individuals had little or no control.[9] In both instances the professional and the health institution proceed from models of health and causality that may not cohere with those of the individuals or groups with whom they work. This practice risks undermining the latter's "subjectivity" or autonomy.[10] The resulting problem can be framed as one of transforming HP/DP practice from "power-over" to "power-with,"[11] and this model has three essential qualities:

1. A noncoercive, dialogic approach to problem naming and problem solving in which both the health professional and the individual or community group presume they have differently useful ways of valuing and understanding health and its determinants;
2. critical reflexivity on the nature of power possessed by people as professionals, and as persons occupying some institutional or bureaucratic position;
3. the exercise of this professional power-over (e.g., authority, status, influence) in ways that strengthen the autonomy of others.

The first quality addresses the issue of how power resides in language and its professional use, such as jargon or labeling, and requires specifying some of the conditions under which professional/client or health system/community group dialogues might be considered noncoercive. Habermas's theory of communicative action offers some help, particularly his idea of an "ideal speech situation" in which people seek an understanding in regard to some practical situation confronting them, by attending to the "validity" of each person's statements: Is it understandable? Does it cohere with empirical accounts? Is its content morally or ethically grounded? Is it spoken with sincerity?[12] The latter two qualities can be illustrated by an example from the Toronto project. "Street" women in a rooming house complained of male residents demanding sexual favors in exchange for access to the bathroom. The women were timid to present their case before the manager and asked a community nurse to speak on their behalf. She did so, using the authority of her professional status to lend credibility to the women's complaints (the second essential quality). But she also informed the women at the outset that they would have to become their own advocates, a role in which she would mentor them (the third essential quality).

Libertarianism's Problematics

Libertarianism must also deal with another *prima facie* health ethics principle, that of justice or creating a "fair distribution of burdens and benefits,"[13] as in my example of improved conditions for women in the house and their ability to negotiate fairer distribution of benefits in the future. But when issues of justice enter a theory of the common good, a narrowly libertarian emphasis on individual autonomy or rights begins to unravel. Theoretically, the libertarian notion of a presocial individual has been criticized for denying the biological "fact" of the mother-child relationship,[14] and by scholars who point to the ways in which ideas of autonomy and individualism only take on meaning in the context of social relationships.[15] But it is in extending the argument of respect for autonomy from dyadic or small group exchanges to larger economic and societal contracts that libertarianism comes under most criticism. For example,

1. Libertarianism's underpinning assumption, namely, that rational choice, even when manifest as collective action,[16] is driven by self-interest conflicts with evidence that many other considerations motivate behavior.[17]

2. The free markets that neoliberal economists and libertarian philosophers claim are most efficient in achieving "the greatest good for the greatest number" necessarily create losers as well as winners, rendering it quite rational for losers to demand some social regulation over the forces that may have victimized them.[18]

3. Even if such markets were truly "free" and operated with textbook perfection, their common good outcomes would still rest on historic inequalities between people and place.[19]

If we accept that any common good notion entails some measure of justice or distributive equity (fairness), libertarian ideas of how it should be achieved have failed the test of history.[20] The past two decades of economic and social policies based on libertarian assumptions, such as privatization of public services, liberalized trade and investment markets, and declining government regulation, have seen wealth inequalities grow to the point where, in the United States and the United Kingdom, they are at their recorded worst.[21] Canada has been the only Organization for Economic Cooperation and Development (OECD) country in the past decade not to experience widening income inequalities, due to redistributive health and social programs and direct income transfers undertaken by the state.[22] Markets are not, in the absence of government interventions, geared to produce a "fair distribution of burdens and benefits," or to guard the sustainability of ecosystems or natural resources.[23]

Recognizing the inevitability of conflict between individual rights, particularly economic rights, and the health or well-being of the larger collective, Canada's *Action Statement* enunciated its second principle: Individual liberties are respected, but priority is given to the common good when conflict arises. This claim positions HP/DP within a social justice, rather than libertarian, theory of the common good, but it begs the question: How do we know when individual liberties conflict with the common good?

Equality of Outcome, Not Equality of Opportunity

In 1986 the World Health Assembly unanimously passed a resolution declaring, in part, that the ultimate goal of development is improved quality of life and well-being for entire national populations, and we will know we are achieving this to the extent that health improves for society's most vulnerable, poorest, and least powerful.[24] This is a teleological ethic, concerned less with the means or duties than with outcomes. Such is the nature of social justice claims. This principle also echoes Aristotle's much older discussion of democracy, through which "the common good for all" is created from public dialogue among people-as-equals. In creating people-as-equals, the democratic state has an obligation to provide "lasting prosperity to the poor by distribution of public revenues," in effect, to function as a welfare state.[25] The common good envisioned here is not one of equality of opportunities, as contemporary debates over social inequalities are often framed, but equality of outcomes. Equality of opportunities is compatible with the libertarian discourse on individual rights and meritocracy. The state's obligation is simply to ensure that everyone has the same opportunity to be considered for a job, invest in the stock market, borrow venture capital from the bank, and so on. After that, let the chips fall where they may. This notion, however, is counterfactual since it rests on ignoring inequalities in resource allocations (by geography, class, sex, or race) based, at least in part, on how the chips fell in earlier rounds. Equality of outcomes, in contrast, has always formed part of the rights or entitlement claims of marginalized or less powerful social groups.

The Common Good in Three Different Health Approaches or Discourses

Giving equality of outcome precedence over equality of opportunity nonetheless raises the question of what we mean by "improved health." In the specific or situated ethics of HP/DP practice, there are at least three explanatory systems for health, each of which might answer this question differently (Table 1). They also offer different constructions of the common good ethical issues facing practice.

The Medical Approach

The common good question in the medical approach can be expressed as the "prevention paradox," in which interventions in cases of pathology show immediate individual results whereas HP/DP health interventions generally do not. This outcome generates public and political support for the former but not for the latter. There is no simple way around this paradox, although when HP/DP programs are posed *against* traditional health care (e.g., in terms of health care cost savings) public support wanes.[26] But public opinion is self-contradictory. People may want traditional health care, and a safe environment, and affordable housing, and more disposable income or lower taxes, and perhaps even more HP/DP programs, without seeing that some choices,

Table 1. Three Different Health Explanatory Systems

	Medical	Behavioral	Socioenvironmental
Define health as	biomedical, absence of disease, disability	medical, plus functional ability, personal wellness, healthy lifestyles	medical and behavioral, plus quality of life, social relationships
Explain health by	pathology, physiological risk factors	medical, plus behavioral risk factors	medical and behavioral plus psychosocial risk factors and socioenvironmental risk conditions
Have different targets for intervention	high-risk individuals	high-risk groups	high-risk conditions
Have different criteria for success	decreased morbidity, age standardized mortality, prevalence of physiological risk factors improved individual QALYs	improved individual lifestyles (behavior change) adoption of healthier lifestyles earlier in "life cycle" decreased population physiological and behavioral risk factors	improved social relationships and networks improved quality of life movement toward social equity (more equal distribution of wealth/power) movement toward environmental sustainability
Variously describe the Common Good Issue	prevention paradox	individual rights *vs.* state utilitarianism	"empowered" relationship between state and communities to create health-promoting conditions

even under conditions of greater distributive equity, cancel out others. The usual way around this problem is to claim that allocations should be based on "needs" rather than "wants,"[27] but this method simply begs the question of who defines "need" and how.[28] Another approach would be to distinguish public opinion from public judgment, the latter being a more deliberative process of arriving at some public choice, not dissimilar from Habermas's theory of communicative action. Under more or less "ideal speech" conditions, and when HP/DP is framed as an extension of health care, public support for such programs becomes stronger.[29]

The Behavioral Approach

The common good question in the behavioral approach rests in the tension between an individual's right to act in personally unhealthy ways (libertarian autonomy) and the state's common good obligation to dissuade or regulate against such choices on the utilitarian grounds that it creates unnecessary risks for others or collective costs and hardships. This is the way in which HP/DP ethics are usually framed.[30] It is also where the social justice argument becomes decidedly murkier. Some cases of common good intervention may be fairly evident, as when nonsmoking workers request or support workplace smoking bans. But many cases are not so evident, as in workplace hiring that discriminates against smokers or programs that monitor employees for tobacco use outside their working hours. Even in "fairly evident" cases there are ethical subtleties, such as when research finds that smoking is being used as stress-coping or as a psychological reward by lower-income single mothers,[31] and so has both positive and negative health effects; that a lifestyle focus on lower social class "target groups" could add to their experience of stress or low self-esteem, causing some degree of health harm; and that the epidemiological construct of risk, locating it as a characteristic of individuals or groups, may create psychologically unhealthy self-identities. There are three ways in which some resolution to the libertarian/communitarian dilemma might be reached:

1. The question should not be posed as one of state intervention for the common good *against* individual liberties. This tactic frames the problem dichotomously rather than opening it to consideration of situations in which the common good should be superordinate. Rather, some reasoned agreement on goals related to the common good should be reached before raising the question of how far its pursuit should override individual liberties.

2. If the question is posed in absolute terms it remains unresolvable. If the question is thought about in more situated or specific practice terms, its contingent resolution becomes easier. Health groups structured around the immediate concerns of lower-income women (such as body image, parenting, managing food budgets) contribute to improved social support, self-esteem and perceived power, creating a context in which self-expressed concerns over smoking or other health behaviors often arise.[32] One could argue that this simply represents a more subtle way of "targeting" behavior change programs for "at risk" groups, but there is a difference: the HP/DP practice is concerned more with the quality of group members' experiences of social relationships and self-identities than with changes in specified health behaviors. Similarly, the City of Toronto some years ago initiated an internal workplace smoking ban as a "test run" for a proposed bylaw. Negotiations between management (which wanted to keep costs low and maintain labor peace), unions (which did not want worker solidarity split by pitting smokers against nonsmokers and which had a more general concern with overall indoor air quality), and the public health department (which wanted to eliminate exposure to environmental tobacco smoke) reframed the issue as one of "no exposure to a known carcinogen" (which all three groups could support). An overhaul of air ventilation systems and testing for other airborne toxins were initiated in addition to a smoking ban.

3. All state action involves some regulation of public life and, despite the notion that most people don't want big government, "polls consistently show that voters want almost all of the big things that big domestic government does."[33] To the extent that HP/DP frames the question of improved health in terms of personal behavior, it is likely to remain locked in the paradigm of state intervention against individual liberties. As my two examples of contingent resolution indicate, support for state interventions on health issues may increase if they are seen as responding, at least in part, to broader health concerns expressed by groups, especially those pertaining more to the quality of social relationships or living and working conditions.

The Socioenvironmental Approach

These broader health concerns comprise the terrain of the third, or socioenvironmental, approach to health, which gained international attention in 1986 with the release of the *Ottawa Charter for Health Promotion*. The *Charter* identified as "health prerequisites" such conditions as "peace . . . income, a stable ecosystem, sustainable resources, social justice and equity."[34] Sometimes dismissed as more ideological than scientific, the *Charter's* concern with social and environmental issues, rather than simply individual behaviors, is supported by a growing body of research evidence, modeled in Figure 1. People living in "risk conditions" structured by economic and political practices have more disease and premature death and less well-being (perceived happiness, quality of life). They often internalize the unfairness of their social circumstances as aspects of their own "badness," thereby increasing their "psychosocial risk factors," which are also associated with poorer health outcomes. This internalization, or self-victimization, is more common when the dominant social discourse on success is competitiveness and meritocracy (people get what they deserve and deserve what they get). Such persons often manifest "behavioral risk factors" partly as coping or reward mechanisms. All of these conditions and factors independently and interdependently increase health-threatening "physiological risk factors."[35] While many health departments and HP/DP practitioners accept risk conditions as health determinants in their own right, others view them more as "holding categories" statistically associated with increased rates of smoking, poor diet, and indolence. These practitioners become interested in poverty not for its own sake, but because poor people smoke more. This embodies social justice to the extent that shorter, more diseased lives attributable to smoking or poor nutrition are considered by HP/DP practitioners and poor people alike to reflect the absence of a common good. But it risks certain health harms and fails to consider the enormity of health inequalities arising from poverty or social inequality independent of health behavior.

Making the Boundaries Permeable

The tension between DP (behavioral risk factors) and HP (risk conditions and psychosocial risk factors) still defines much HP/DP practice. Even Canada's *Action Statement* was self-critical on the extent to which lifestyle health issues still dominate practice. But the resolution is not to set health behaviors against risk conditions or to simply see conditions as determinants of behavior or, "predisposing factors," as they are called in Green and Kreuter's influential modeling.[36] Instead, there are two tasks a socioenvironmental approach poses for a politics of practice. The first task, as the Toronto health department argues in one of its policy reports, is to

> . . . continuously seek to intervene at the level of psychosocial risk factor or risk condition. Department staff encounter a myriad of individual

Health Determinants

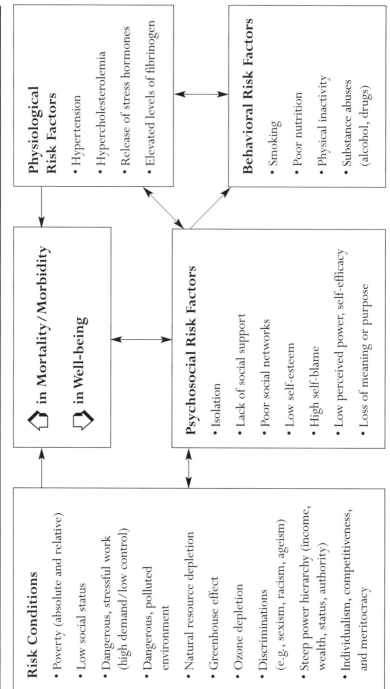

Risk Conditions

- Poverty (absolute and relative)
- Low social status
- Dangerous, stressful work (high demand/low control)
- Dangerous, polluted environment
- Natural resource depletion
- Greenhouse effect
- Ozone depletion
- Discriminations (e.g, sexism, racism, ageism)
- Steep power hierarchy (income, wealth, status, authority)
- Individualism, competitiveness, and meritocracy

Psychosocial Risk Factors

- Isolation
- Lack of social support
- Poor social networks
- Low self-esteem
- High self-blame
- Low perceived power, self-efficacy
- Loss of meaning or purpose

⬆ in Mortality / Morbidity

⬇ in Well-being

Physiological Risk Factors

- Hypertension
- Hypercholesterolemia
- Release of stress hormones
- Elevated levels of fibrinogen

Behavioral Risk Factors

- Smoking
- Poor nutrition
- Physical inactivity
- Substance abuses (alcohol, drugs)

problems in their work. The socioenvironmental approach requires that we look for patterns in these individual problems and begin to think of them in terms of social issues, and that we seek to remedy them with collective action.[37]

The second task becomes one of "making the boundaries permeable" among the medical, behavioral, and socioenvironmental approaches.[38] One heart health project, for example, found that organizing in a poor neighborhood was easier around "one-off" community picnics, fun runs and collective dinners than around more complex problems of poverty, unemployment, or housing. But, over time, community members on the heart health organizing committee began to raise these more systemic concerns. Rather than worrying that these issues were outside their heart health mandate, practitioners instead examined how they and their health department could support the group's organizing efforts on these more difficult problems.[39]

Funding programs for substance abuse and AIDS prevention administered by the Toronto health department also adopted a socioenvironmental approach to these problems, which allowed them to support various forms of community organizing and political education projects only indirectly concerned with either drugs or AIDS. But a socioenvironmental approach can be so broad in scope that it fails to provide guidance to health systems attempting to make allocative decisions under conditions of competing community demands. The department's resolution was not to retreat to more narrowly defined behavioral objectives, but to meet annually with interested community groups to negotiate issue and strategy priorities for each funding round.[40] (These examples also illustrate other transformative uses of professionals' and health systems' socially structured power-over).

Social Justice's Problematics

The emphasis of a socioenvironmental approach on using public policy to create health-promoting conditions raises two new problematics with a social justice theory of the common good. The first relates to how HP/DP practitioners perceive the relative responsibility of the state and communities for achieving common good objectives. The health sector is not alone in this. As social inequalities widen in the wake of the dominant libertarian discourse and its sequella of market deregulation and welfare state minimalism, discussions of civil society, social capital, and communitarianism are on the upsurge in both academic and popular media. Despite criticisms that these concepts tend to be undertheorized and oversimplified,[41] they speak to a growing public disenchantment with libertarianism's "selfish ethos."[42] One might even suggest that the language of civil society or social capital, or "the restoration of community," is where an HP/DP common good ought to locate itself, and many writers, notably Amitai Etzioni, directly or indirectly have done so.[43] Certainly, the language of "strengthening communities" suffused many recent HP/DP normative claims and is evident in its research focus on such constructs as "community empowerment" and "community capacity."

Without minimizing the contribution voluntary associational memberships can make to health and social justice, there are several problems with a narrow communitarian formulation of the common good which, ironically, align it more with libertarianism:

1. It implies community or civil society properties of nonconflictive cohesiveness that it does not possess.
2. It underplays the role governments have in *constituting* civil society, or at least its possibilities, including evidence that government-initiated neighborhood associations or citizen bodies sometimes "outperform" strictly voluntary bodies,[44] and that the institutionalization of voluntary groups brought on by partnerships with government can broaden groups' goals and enhance their internal democracy "while maintaining a sense of community that allow[s] [groups] to resist cooptation."[45]
3. It ignores the historical role played by government social or welfare policies in creating conditions supportive to the cause of many marginalized groups (women, ethnic or racial minorities, gays and lesbians, and so on).
4. It tends to be silent on the two great social phenomena of our era: globalization of commerce, in which the erosion of social capital is due not to citizen withdrawal from voluntarism and good works but to private capital's withdrawal from any civic duty, and the consequent and steady decline in the "fair distributive" role of the welfare state.[46]

Not all writers on communitarianism or civic society have ignored these issues, and a more sophisticated conceptualization of the role of the state in mediating between differently powered "interest groups" in society or, in political economy terms, between markets and communities, is slowly reemerging.[47] A social justice theory of the common good, then, at least as it pertains to the situated practice of HP/DP, would organize itself around two questions:

1. How does the relationship between state institutions, particularly health systems, and community groups further progress (act) toward the creation of more health-promoting conditions?
2. What specifically do HP/DP practitioners and health systems contribute to this progress?

Participatory Relationships: A Theory of Deliberative Democracy

The first of these two questions raises the other problematic with a social justice theory, that of how common good policies are publicly determined. As another of the *Action Statement's* principles argues: "Participation is supported in policy decision-making to identify what constitutes the common good." This does not reduce definition of the common good to a relativist mishmash of claims but emphasizes again the importance of a dialogic relationship between health systems and community members. Drugs, for example, are often cited as a leading concern in many poorer communities. But there are many ways in which the "drug problem" might be understood, for example, in terms of physical addiction, crime, lack of awareness, or lack of future opportunity. Each of these analytical maps, while not necessarily exclusive, would yield different HP/DP interventions. Only in a critical and reflective dialogue with community residents can HP/DP practitioners determine the most useful "map" to guide their programs.[48]

This dialogic relationship is nothing other than a restatement of democracy. Lester Thurow's argument that the dominant American values of libertarianism and democracy "have no 'common good'" but "stress the individual and not the group,"[49] may be the case with libertarianism but applies to democracy only in its "one person, one vote" representational meaning. There is also a long history and intellectual elaboration of participatory democracy that emphasizes the role of collectivities of actors in political participation. John Gardner has cautioned that this vision of messy political jockeying can, "without commitment to the common good," become "a pluralism gone berserk."[50] One can as easily argue, however, that this contingent politicking is necessary to *define* the specifics of the common good and, to the extent that it is deliberative, critical, and reflective, actually *represents* a common good. But these features of deliberation, critique, and reflection are essential; without them, participatory democracy becomes little other than a contest between unequals where the historically more powerful prevail.

Amy Gutmann, in an essay that reconciles libertarianism's emphasis on autonomy with democracy's crude "majoritarianism," cautions against a simplistic concept of participatory democracy as one in which "a polity . . . all actively make decisions."[51] This state is unachievable except for the small, romanticized communities envisioned by Etzioni's communitarianism. Instead, Gutmann elaborates a theory of "deliberative democracy," characterized by "an ideal of politics" where people routinely relate to one another "by influencing each other through the publicly valued use of reasoned argument, evidence, evaluation, and persuasion that enlists reason in its cause," an ideal not dissimilar from that of Habermas's theory of communicative action. She goes on to argue that

> Accountability, not direct participation, is the key to deliberative democracy. Accountability is a form of active political engagement, but it does not require continual and direct involvement in politics; it is fully compatible with the division of labor between professional politicians and citizens that is characteristic of representative democracy.[52]

This "compatibility" fits well with actual, rather than ideal, accounts of effective citizen participation, in which there is only occasional direct participation between state institutions and citizen (community) groups on issues of substantive importance.[53] Deliberative democracy does not preclude direct participation; it merely puts limits around it. Individuals and groups can seek to influence those who make decisions on their behalf and, at minimum, have a moral obligation to ensure that such persons are accountable to those they claim to represent. Part of this accountability rests on the reciprocating obligations of public and political institutions to become more transparent in their operations and "to help citizens make well-informed decisions about their collective life, enlisting their critical capacities in making political choices."[54] This theory of democracy offers no absolutist "calculus of choice," and accepts the "disharmony" that democratic deliberation necessarily entails. At base, it rests upon "institutions that support public deliberation and accountability on matters of political importance."[55] This may seem an unrealistic ideal, at least at senior state levels where money and social status often define what is of political importance. But there are numerous examples of genuine efforts at such deliberation, albeit often at more local levels; and, within the health sector, it has often been the rhetoric of HP/DP that has helped to prod institutions in this direction.[56]

Overcoming Historic Exclusion

There remains one more problem that must be overcome with a theory of the common good that incorporates a democratic ideal simultaneously embracing representational and deliberative/participatory norms. How does it confront social forces that exclude less powerful groups from both forms of democratic expression or, as David Richards expressed, how does it overcome sexism and racism as "historically powerful communities of thought and practice" that "have allowed no space for the equal participation of woman [and nondominant ethnic or racial groups] . . . in the deliberative discourse about justice and public and personal good"?[57] This is where a social justice concern with equality of outcome conflicts with the libertarian concern with equality of opportunity, for, as another of the *Action Statement's* principles reads: "Priority is given to people whose living conditions, especially a lack of wealth and power, place them at greater risk."

Equality of outcome in the face of historic exclusion requires inequality of opportunity. This argument is not a popular one in today's libertarian-inspired backlash against various reverse discrimination or affirmative action programs. It is nonetheless defensible when considering what we know about traditional barriers to political and policy participation by poorer groups, such as resource constraints and acculturated beliefs and behaviors that condition their apathy and politicians to align with the interests of elite groups.[58] Occasionally the policy call for targeting public health or HP/DP resources to particular groups is challenged on the basis that such programs should be universal. Certainly, there are powerful arguments in favor of universal health and social programs over means-tested or targeted programs. Universality helps to build social solidarity and, pragmatically, increases support for "well/fair" programs. (I thank Alex Scott-Samuel of Liverpool University for this clever play on words.) Any distributive inequality that might arise from universality (e.g., high-income families have less need for child benefit transfers or educational deductions) can be dealt with through progressive forms of income or consumption taxation. But even within universal programs, health systems and practitioners are constantly making situational choices over who gets first or most attention, and who does not. In emergency rooms, these triage decisions are based on estimates of physiological need or urgency. In HP/DP work, these triage decisions would be based on estimates of psychosocial or political legitimacy/resource mobilization needs or urgency and, in a more general sense, on which individuals or groups would assist most in creating more health-promoting conditions.

Recognizing that any decision to work with one group perforce implies a decision not to work with others helps to overcome the prevention paradox discussed earlier. Medical interventions invariably involve decisions that favor one person or problem over another. Except under idealized conditions of perfect markets, health care is and has always been rationed. The same situation applies to HP/DP. Apart from social marketing or education campaigns targeting specific behavioral risk factors, HP/DP practice does afford immediate benefits to particular individuals or groups, usually in the form of material, financial, or human resources, or improved political legitimacy. When HP/DP practice helps to organize or mobilize groups, benefits in terms of enhanced social support, self-efficacy, or renewed meaning and purpose also arise, even if the group "fails" to win particular social campaigns for health-promoting policy changes. To the extent that support to these groups is useful to their work, HP/DP practitioners and health systems have public allies in defense of their programs. What remains troublesome for health systems, however, is that the "products" of this work are rarely measurable in terms of morbidity or mortality rates, have different program objectives than conventional medical or behavioral approaches, and may not be easily quantifiable. This is a long-standing issue in the literature on HP/DP evaluation, but its elaboration lies beyond this paper's purview. Still, health systems administrators concerned with accountability of a social justice oriented HP/DP practice should keep this important point in mind. Research, such as that cited in support of the health determinants model in Figure 1, illuminates the linkages between risk conditions, psychosocial risk factors, health behaviors, physiological impacts and, ultimately, death and disease and perceived well-being. HP/DP programs rarely have the resources or capacity to demonstrate these links with any degree of rigor. Our health systems do not demand that each case of heart surgery demonstrates its impact on aggregate health status, only that the patient does not needlessly die, experiences an improved quality of life, and that the procedure follows accepted norms of practice. The same applies to HP/DP programs, which, though they should be accountable for actions associated with improved health, are deemed sufficient if they do not needlessly harm the health or well-being of individuals involved in the program, do improve the immediate quality of life for participants, and are consistent with accepted norms of practice.

Conclusion: Toward a Practice of Deliberative Democracy

In this chapter I reviewed two major theories of the common good: libertarianism and its emphasis on individual autonomy, and social justice and its emphasis on the collectivity. While libertarianism offers helpful cautions against the tendency of state institutions to power-over individuals and their capacity for reasoned reflection and choice, its extension to political and economic relations in the form of weak state interventions and "free" economic markets conflicts with evidence that strong state interventions are required to regulate markets to achieve living and working conditions that are health promoting. A social justice theory, by contrast, is consistent with evidence on the centrality of economic equality and environmental sustainability to public health and with international health accords that position equality in outcome as a superordinate ethic to equality in opportunity. I discussed how movement toward equality in outcome might differ according to the assumptions underpinning three different approaches to HP/DP: the medical, behavioral, and socioenvironmental. I cautioned on both ethical and practical grounds that HP/DP practice needs to

1. position itself as an extension of traditional health care (the medical approach), rather than against it;
2. avoid dichotomous debates around lifestyles that become absolutist and unresolvable, rather than contingent and negotiable;
3. posit common good goals before considering the extent to which "society" is willing to accept regulatory curtailments on individual liberties for their achievement;
4. extend its range of concern to incorporate risk conditions and psychosocial risk factors, which are often of greater importance to less powerful or poorer community groups.

In doing so, and to avoid slipping into a naive language of communitarianism, the situated practice of HP/DP must become more critically reflective on how relationships between state or state-funded health institutions and groups in civil society might become more empowering, in the sense of engendering more action toward the creation of health-promoting conditions. I argued for improved and relevant forms of citizen participation in public policymaking, and in particular for a deliberative approach to democracy based on principles of reasoned argument, evidence, and evaluation, and transparency, openness, and accountability in public institutions. Only in this way can the more contingent policy objectives consistent with movement toward equality of outcomes be negotiated with the people who will be affected by them. But equality of outcome requires inequality of opportunity. To be consistent with a social justice theory of the common good, HP/DP practice must counter the traditional forces that exclude nonelite groups from this democratic deliberation. It must, therefore, at least in part, target certain groups or issues for support and action, even within the context of nominally universal programs.

Throughout, I have formulated only a few broad principles for a social justice oriented HP/DP practice, eschewing any absolute theory or ethic of the common good in support of one that is continuously skeptical of "final" accounts and subject to ongoing public dialogue and judgment. My arguments might be criticized for their normative quality, although I attempted to illustrate at least some of them with examples from practice. Practice, of course, is more modest in its effect than the claims of philosophy and political theory. But it is at the more mundane level of how people treat each other that civic society and a common good are created and bases established for collective actions at higher political levels. Democracy, whether representative, participatory, or deliberative, is like power. It cannot be given, only taken. It is something that must be affirmed and struggled for on a daily basis.

NOTES

1. D. Smith, "Geography, Health and Social Justice: Looking for the 'Right' Theory," *Critical Public Health* 6, no. 3 (1995): 5–11.

2. Ronald Labonte, "Population Health and Health Promotion: What Do They Have to Say to Each Other?" *Canadian Journal of Public Health* 86, no. 3 (1995): 165–68.

3. Canadian Public Health Association, *Action Statement on Health Promotion in Canada* (Ottawa: Author, 1996).

4. Ann Pederson and Louise Signal, "The Health Promotion Movement in Ontario: Mobilizing to Broaden the Definition of Health," in *Health Promotion in Canada,* ed. Ann Pederson, Michel O'Neill, and Irv Rootman (Toronto: W. B. Saunders, 1994).

5. P. Duncan and A. Cribb, "Helping People Change: An Ethical Approach?" *Health Education Research* 11, no. 3 (1996): 339–48.

6. M. Bloor and J. McIntosh, "Surveillance and Concealment," in *Readings in Medical Sociology,* ed. Sarah Cunningham-Burley and Neil McKeganey (New York: Tavistock/Routledge, 1990); G. Scambler, "Habermas and the Power of Medical Expertise," in *Sociological Theory and Medical Sociology,* ed. G. Scambler (New York: Methuen, 1987).

7. Nina Wallerstein, "Powerlessness, Empowerment and Health: Implications for Health Promotion Programs," *American Journal of Health Promotion* 6, no. 3 (1992): 197–205.

8. Labonte, "Health Promotion and Empowerment: Reflections on Professional Practice," *Health Education Quarterly* 21, no. 2 (1994): 253–68.

9. Labonte and Susan Penfold, "Canadian Perspectives in Health Promotion: a Critique," *Health Education* 19 (1981): 4–9.

10. W. Hollway, "Gender Difference and the Production of Subjectivity," in *Changing the Subject: Psychology, Social Regulation and Subjectivity,* ed. J. Henriques et al. (London: Methuen, 1984).

11. Meredith Minkler, "Introduction and Overview," in *Community Organizing and Community Building for Health* (London: Rutgers University Press, 1997) pp. 3–19; Labonte, "Community Development in the Public Health Sector: The Possibilities of an Empowering Relationship between State and Civil Society" (Ph.D. diss., York University, 1996).

12. Juergen Habermas, *The Theory of Communicative Action,* vol. 1 (London: Heinemann, 1984).

13. R. Purtilo, *Ethical Dimensions in the Health Professions* (Toronto: W. B. Saunders, 1981).

14. M. Ferree, "The Political Context of Rationality: Rational Choice and Resource Mobilization Theory," in *Frontiers in Social Movement Theory,* ed. A. Morriss and C. Meuller (New Haven: Yale University Press, 1992); J. Tronto, *Moral Boundaries: A Political Argument for an Ethic of Care* (New York: Routledge, 1993).

15. S. Seidman and D. Wagner, eds., *Postmodernism and Social Theory* (Oxford: Blackwell, 1992).

16. Mancur Olson, *The Logic of Collective Action: Public Goods and the Theory of Groups* (Boston: Harvard University Press, 1965).

17. David Knoke, *Organizing for Collective Action* (New York: Aldine de Gruyter, 1990).

18. R. Dahl, "Why All Democratic Countries Have Mixed Economies," in *Democratic Community,* ed. J. Chapman and I. Shapiro, Nomos 35 (New York: New York University Press, 1993), pp. 259–82.

19. Smith, "Geography, health."

20. R. Boyer and D. Drache, introduction to *States Against Market: The Limits of Globalization,* ed. R. Boyer and D. Drache (New York: Routledge,

1996); R. Burbach, O. Nunez, and B. Kagarlitsky, *Globalization and Its Discontents* (London: Polity Press, 1997).

21. Public Citizens Global Trade Watch Backgrounder, "The Alarming Multilateral Agreement on Investment" http://www.islandnet.com/plethora/maibg.html, 1997; Robert Reich, "The Missing Options," *American Prospect* 35 (1997): 6–13.

22. National Forum on Health, *Canada's Health Action: Building on the Legacy* (Ottawa: Author, 1997).

23. Herman Daly and John Cobb, *For the Common Good* (Boston: Beacon Press, 1989).

24. World Health Assembly, "The Role of Intersectoral Cooperation in National Strategies for Health for All," *Health Promotion* 1, no. 2 (1986): 239–51.

25. Noam Chomsky, "The Common Good," http://www.islandnet.com/plethora/chomsky2.html, 1997.

26. National Forum on Health, *Canada's Health Action.*

27. D. Seedhouse and L. Lovett, *Practical Medical Ethics* (Chichester, U.K.: John Wiley, 1992).

28. Nancy Fraser, *Unruly Practices: Power Discourse and Gender in Contemporary Social Theory* (Minneapolis, Minn.: University of Minnesota Press, 1989).

29. National Forum on Health, *Canada's Health Action.*

30. Duncan and Cribb, "Helping People Change."

31. Hilary Graham, "Women's Smoking and Family Health," *Social Science and Medicine* 1 (1987): 47–56.

32. Marjorie Kort, *Turning Point: A Health Promotion Demonstration Project* (Ottawa: Centretown Community Health Centre and South East Ottawa Community Resource Centre, 1990).

33. J. Faux, "Can Liberals Tell a Credible Story?" *American Prospect* 35 (1997): 28–33.

34. World Health Organization, *Ottawa Charter for Health Promotion* (Copenhagen: Author, 1986).

35. Labonte, *Power, Participation and Partnerships* (Melbourne: VicHealth Foundation, 1997).

36. L. Green and M. Kreuter, *Health Promotion Planning: An Educational and Environmental Approach* (Mountain View, Calif.: Mayfield, 1991).

37. Toronto Department of Public Health, *Advocacy for Basic Health Prerequisites* (Toronto: Department of Public Health, 1991).

38. Labonte, *Community Development.*

39. Labonte and Ann Robertson, "Health Promotion Research and Practice: The Case for the Constructivist Paradigm," *Health Education Quarterly* 26, no. 4 (1996): 431–47.

40. Labonte, "Community Development."

41. M. Foley and B. Edwards, "Escape from Politics? Social theory and the Social Capital Debate," *American Behavioral Scientist* 40, no. 5 (1997): 550–61.

42. Michael Lerner, *The Politics of Meaning: Restoring Hope and Possibility in an Age of Cynicism* (Don Mills: Addison-Wesley, 1996); M. Minkler and C. Pies, "Ethical Issues in Community Organization and Community Participation," in *Community Organizing and Community Building for Health,* ed. M. Minkler (London: Rutgers University Press, 1997), pp. 120–38.

43. John McKnight, "Regenerating Community," *Social Policy* (Winter 1987): 54–58; Amitai Etzioni, *The Spirit of Community* (Toronto: Simon and Schuster, 1993).

44. K. Portney and J. Berry, "Social Capital and Participation in Urban Neighbourhoods," *American Behavioral Scientist* 40, no. 5 (1997): 632–44.

45. C. Siriani, "Learning Pluralism: Democracy and Diversity in Feminist Organizations," in *Democratic Community,* ed. J. Chapman and I. Shapiro, Nomos 35 (New York: New York University Press, 1993), pp. 283–312.

46. Edwards and Foley, "Social Capital and the Political Economy of Our Discontent," *American Behavioral Scientist* 40, no. 5 (1997): 669–78.

47. I. Culpitt, *Welfare and Citizenship: Beyond the Crisis of the Welfare State* (London: Sage, 1992); C. Pierson, *Beyond the Welfare State?* (London: Polity Press, 1994); T. Skocpol, "The Potential Autonomy of the State," in *Power in Modern Societies,* ed. M. Olsen and M. Marger (San Francisco: Westview Press, 1993); F. Twine, *Citizenship and Social Rights: The Interdependence of Self and Society* (London: Sage, 1994).

48. Toronto Department of Public Health, *Making Communities* (Toronto: Department of Public Health, 1994).

49. Lester Thurow, *The Future of Capitalism* (New York: William Morrow, 1966).

50. John Gardner, *Building Communities* (Stanford University: Independent Sector Leadership Studies Program, 1991).

51. Amy Gutmann, "The Disharmony of Democracy," in *Democratic Community,* ed. J. Chapman and I. Shapiro, Nomos 35 (New York: New York University Press, 1993), pp. 126–62.

52. Gutmann, "The Disharmony," p. 143.

53. Labonte and Rick Edwards, *Equity in Action: Supporting the Public in Public Policy* (Toronto: Centre for Health Promotion/Participation, 1995).

54. Gutmann, "The Disharmony," p. 148.

55. Gutmann, "The Disharmony," p. 150.

56. Labonte, "Community Development."

57. David Richards, "Political Theory and the Aims of Feminism," in *Democratic Community,* ed. J. Chapman and I. Shapiro, Nomos 35 (New York: New York University Press, 1993), pp. 414–22.

58. Labonte and Edwards, *Equity in Action.*

BARBARA A. KOENIG AND ALAN STOCKDALE

The Promise of Molecular Medicine in Preventing Disease: Examining the Burden of Genetic Risk

As many undoubtedly know, we are about half-way through a major scientific enterprise: the effort to map and sequence the full human genome.[1] By early next century the complete compliment of human genes will be readily available to researchers; the known associations between diseases and genotypes will climb geometrically. The new "molecular" medicine offers great promise in many areas of health care, including the prevention of disease in those believed to be "at risk." In this chapter we provide a brief outline of the implications of advances in the genomic sciences for disease prevention and health promotion.

We argue that the concept of risk, so central to work in public health, has clear but unrecognized burdens associated with it. Identification of susceptibility genes for common illnesses such as cancer and coronary heart disease will highlight those burdens.[2] We pay special attention to the unexamined "claims" of prevention practices. One of those claims is that risk is a technical, scientific category, unsullied by cultural, social, or political forces. Another claim is that clear benefits accrue from the precise calculation of disease "risk" and its assignment to certain individuals or groups. What are the unexamined costs associated with the risk language so ubiquitous in public health practice? How will those costs be intensified by the increasing power of the genetic paradigm in health promotion and disease prevention?

As anthropologists working within the interdisciplinary field of bioethics and specializing in the cultural analysis of scientific biomedicine, we take as a general rule the need to question the face value of the terms and concepts underlying our everyday health practices. We see our principal task to be "investigating the processes by which certain forms of knowledge achieve legitimacy and appear to be part of the natural order."[3] For that reason, we begin our analysis by making the term "risk" itself "problematic," examining the cultural assumptions underlying the risk "discourse" that is so pervasive in contemporary health care. We will have been successful if at the end of this chapter the reader finds him or herself unable to use the term "risk" without a moment's questioning and hesitation.

In making our argument we use clinical examples from the evolving field of genetic medicine, however, we emphasize one case example, the developing technology of predisposition genetic testing—sometimes called susceptibility testing—for breast and ovarian cancer.[4] We only have space to provide a brief introduction to the genetics of breast cancer.[5] For readers unfamiliar with this particularly dramatic case study of molecular genetic medicine, it has recently been established that mutations in two genes, named BRCA1 and BRCA2, account for most of the 5 to 10 percent of breast cancer that is believed to be inherited. A commercial test for BRCA1/2 alterations is available. Thus, genetic testing for breast cancer susceptibility ("risk") is one of the first widely available tests for a common adult-onset disease. It is also a molecular test for a disease that has not traditionally been understood to be of genetic origin. Testing for BRCA1/2 mutations represents a new phenomenon: the expansion of a genetic mode of explanation to new categories of illness.

A mutation in one of the newly identified breast cancer genes is thought to raise a woman's lifetime risk of breast cancer to approximately 70 to 85 percent, compared with the average, or population risk for women of about 9 percent over a lifetime. These mutations, especially BRCA1, are also associated with increased risk of ovarian cancer, which is estimated to range from approximately 15 to 45 percent for carriers of BRCA1 by age seventy.[6] Unfortunately, once tested and identified as being "at risk," there is little that a woman can do to prevent the onset of cancer. Recent studies of chemoprevention drugs suggest that this approach offers potential benefit, although this is as yet unproven in the situation of heightened genetic susceptibility to breast cancer. Other than dramatic surgeries to remove the breasts or ovaries, the only option women currently have is the frequent use of standard disease screening practices, such as mammography and breast self-exam. Early detection strategies for ovarian cancer are of even less certain value, and preventive technologies do not exist.

Our primary message is that the concept of risk, and in particular genetic risk, is extremely problematic. At one level risk is a neutral, scientific term that can be specified with mathematical certainty. A technical definition of the term is "an adverse future event that is not certain but only probable."[7] However, as we hope to make clear, the social implications of a public health discourse based on an ever more precise elaboration of risk are profound. As Petersen and Lupton note, "Strict adherence to self-care regimes is seen as the only real means of avoiding the cancers, heart diseases and other afflictions that constantly threaten the integrity of the self in a generalized climate of risk."[8] Understanding the strength of the risk discourse requires an analysis of the cultural forces that shape our response to the uncertainties of disease and bodily deterioration.

The Promise of Molecular Genetics

An editorial in an issue of the *Journal of the American Medical Association* devoted to genetics suggests a future transformed by the use of molecular techniques in prevention: "Imagine a physician discussing the results of a blood test with a patient that shows the risk of colon cancer to be increased four-fold and the risk for diabetes as twice normal. After discussing the meaning of the tests, the physician, the patient, and the nurse design a preventive medicine program to maximize the patient's chances of staying well. This scenario may not be as farfetched or far off as it may seem."[9] The promise of targeted disease prevention based on risk stratification is clearly laid out by Francis Collins, the director of the National Human Genome Research Institute at the U.S. National Institutes of Health. But note the imprecision of language in Collins's quote—"a blood test . . . shows *the* risk of colon cancer . . . *the* risk for diabetes . . . [emphasis added]." It is hard to tell *where* exactly the risk of disease is located. Is it within the individual patient's body or does it reside more accurately as an abstraction derived from a population database? What are the ramifications of locating risk within individual bodies?

The implication of Collins's statement appears to be that the test shows the patient to have a higher than average risk derived from an index population. But how are these figures derived? In the case of classic Mendelian genetic diseases it is often possible to make fairly accurate predictions of future disease occurrence based on knowledge derived from a genetic test because the association between genotype and phenotype is *relatively* simple and the mechanism of inheritance fairly well understood. For example, in the case of Huntington disease, a late-onset disease caused by an autosomal dominant gene, the penetrance of the disease is thought to be close to 100 percent. Thus a person with a mutated or abnormal copy of the Huntington gene will develop the disease provided he or she lives long enough (the uncertainty is primarily in the timing). In the case of the common, generally more complex, diseases, the mechanisms of genetic causation are at present not well understood. The implications of having a BRCA1 or 2 allele associated with breast cancer are unclear, since some women escape cancer in spite of established genetic susceptibility, perhaps because of unknown gene-environment or gene-gene interactions. Furthermore, the figures calculating disease risk over a lifetime are drawn from specific populations. The population may or may not be truly representative of the individual undergoing testing.

Another example of the complexity of drawing associations between genotype and disease is the ApoE allele associated with Alzheimer's disease.[10] In this case there is a correlation between the presence of particular alleles and the incidence of the disease in a given population. Problems arise when a jump is made from risk figures for populations to risk figures for individuals because the various factors that make a particular individual susceptible to the disease in question, and the mechanisms by which they function, are not sufficiently known. Thus, having an allele associated with a disease of this sort does not *necessarily* mean that one will develop the disease or even that one has an above average risk of developing the disease (the "risk" could be revised up or down as more is discovered). Thus the meaning of being "at genetic risk" is quite different in the situation of Huntington disease than in the case of breast cancer or Alzheimer's disease.

What is new in this mode of genetic explanation? Genetic technologies have, of course, been deployed in public health for decades, traditionally in newborn screening programs for genetic illnesses, such as phenylketonuria (PKU) or hypothyroidism. What is new in the scenario presented by Dr. Collins is the focus on common, "polygenic," multifactorial conditions such as cancer, heart disease, and diabetes. A working group at the U.S. Centers for Disease Control and Prevention recently outlined how genetics fits in with traditional understandings of primary, secondary, and tertiary prevention.[11] An example of primary prevention is the discovery of a link between folic acid intake during pregnancy and neural tube defects, a finding that has led to the recommendation that various food products be fortified with folic acid. (There is a related but reverse example—genetic tests may also identify individuals with hemochromatosis, in which people who might be *harmed* by ingestion of iron-fortified foods, a practice meant to improve overall health and eliminate iron deficiency.) Secondary prevention targets clinical manifestations of disease by early detection and intervention during the preclinical phase of the disease. The newborn screening programs are good examples of secondary prevention; in the case of screening for PKU or galactosemia, the intervention involves modifying the effect of a metabolic genetic "error" through diet. Tertiary prevention in genetics minimizes the effects of existing disease by preventing complications or further deterioration. The example given by the CDC group is the use of prophylactic antibiotics for young children with sickle cell anemia.

The Working Group also forecasts a new paradigm of primary prevention. They argue that since many known (nongenetic) risk factors for chronic disease have low predictive value, the use of genetic tests for susceptibility genes may improve the *predictive* value of *environmental* risk factors. Thus the new paradigm in prevention will be the identification and interruption of environmental cofactors that lead to clinical disease among people with susceptibility genes.[12] This hope of individually targeted prevention was suggested by Francis Collins in his *JAMA* editorial. Breast cancer genes provide a good example of this new paradigm. Having a mutation in BRCA1 or 2 does not guarantee that cancer will develop. However, when the right (or wrong) environmental condition interacts with a nonfunctioning BRCA1 or 2 gene—a gene thought to function as a tumor suppresser gene—cancer develops. Perhaps an environmental intervention, such as a modification in diet or reduction in exposure to an occupational hazard, would effectively prevent cancer in those with a mutated gene, whereas it would not be a useful prevention strategy for the entire population. It should be noted that this new paradigm for preventive medicine is not undisputed. Some biologists argue that the assumption that there are discrete genetic and environmental factors that can be added up in a meaningful way is wrongheaded because many complex traits may involve interactive systems that cannot usefully be treated as additive.[13]

The new paradigm may require other changes in thinking. The knowledge gained by genetics and genetic diagnosis will likely break down traditional thinking about the boundaries between prevention and early detection, particularly in cancer. Richard Klausner, the director of the National Cancer Institute, has asked, "If you could detect the earliest genetic changes in a single cell that might lead to cancer many years down the road, and somehow reverse that change or isolate the cell, is that treatment or prevention? Is the affected individual ill or merely at risk? Where do you draw the line?"[14]

Another somewhat ironic feature of the CDC model is the following: Certain genotypes are known to be protective. Some individuals are at lower than average risk for acquiring HIV disease in spite of "exposure," and in another example, certain people are less likely to develop lung cancer, even if they smoke. Risk stratification raises profound questions about egalitarian public health interventions targeted broadly at populations. Should certain people be exempted from public health campaigns, for example campaigns for "safer sex" or smoking cessation programs, because they are deemed to be at low risk? Would people found to be at low risk be informed of their status and be treated differently by their physicians and others? And what would the consequences of the resulting differentiation of genetic subgroups be for the goals of population-based health programs?

The vast amount of genetic information generated by the Human Genome Project will lead to a *qualitative* as well as a purely *quantitative* difference in our ability to customize and individualize disease prevention activities throughout a broad spectrum of public health and clinical practices. The possibility exists that every aspect of clinical practice will be customized. To give a few examples: We can already predict an individual's response to antiretroviral drug therapy for HIV by genotyping the AIDS virus. Similarly, tumors can be genotyped for virulence. For example, in 1998 the Food and Drug Administration approved a gene test to aid the prediction of breast cancer recurrence based on work that associated the overexpression of the HER-2/neu gene with poor clinical outcome in a subset of breast cancer patients.[15] The latter two examples represent the use of genetic data and risk stratification in tertiary disease prevention programs.

Each scientific advance seems to be accompanied by an ethical concern. Do individuals with a poorer prognosis based on an assessment of genetic risk—for example, a prognosis derived from genotyping a tumor—warrant less aggressive (and hence less expensive) treatment? It has long been known that certain individuals are more or less likely to suffer serious side effects from particular drugs or from toxic work environments. An interesting example is the association of a particular genetic variation in the blood's clotting system, called Factor V (Leiden variation).[16] Found in about 3 percent of the population, it may predispose a person to life-threatening venous thrombosis. Should women be screened for this Factor V variant before taking oral contraceptives, a drug known to be associated with clotting disorders? An enormous range of drugs—preventive and curative—will be targeted to individual genetic variation. The very mechanism of drug design and discovery has already been transformed in a few years by the genomics revolution.

To keep the discussion focused and to avoid classificatory issues, we are only using examples of prevention based on risk stratification for conditions commonly and unproblematically understood to be diseases, such as cancer, AIDS, or serious blood disorders. The situation gets much more complicated if we add risk stratification of individuals based on genetic testing for traits such as obesity or conditions like alcoholism with a strong behavioral component. In these cases the moral dimension of claiming genetic risk is even more profound.

The Value of Cultural Analysis

Now that we have provided a very brief synopsis of the promise of molecular genetics in disease prevention, what are the perils, the ethical and social dilemmas? The clinical scenarios described above all share a common feature: in order to target disease prevention or health promotion interventions, individuals must be stratified according to genetic risk. Is risk stratification risky? What are the cultural sources of the need for such levels of control, precision, and certainty?

The *New York Times* science reporter Gina Kolata recently characterized the bioethics community as a "Greek chorus of professional naysayers."[17] Indeed, a veritable industry has grown up devoted to commenting on the ethical, legal, and social implications of advances in human genetic medicine and the genomic sciences. However, although we have been a part of that enterprise, in general we find most of the commentary to be quite narrow, focusing on a few "dangers," primarily insurance and workplace discrimination and the potential for stigmatization. In the health policy world the issues are framed against a background discussion of needed legal reform, as if all that is needed are a few new laws so that science can move forward unimpeded and lives can be saved with new technologies.

In the world of the clinic, concerns about the use of genetic technologies have also been narrowly framed. In this arena the concern is first, with the precise psychological measurement of the impact of genetic testing, for example, how much does depression and anxiety increase (or decrease) when individuals are tested for mutations in the BRCA1 gene and informed of their results? Considering that a young woman's entire view of her future life may be transformed by the risk knowledge transmitted by a BRCA1/2 test, scores on a depression scale seem to be a trivial reflection of the impact of testing. A second concern, one that we would also define as quite narrow, is the impact of genetic knowledge on surveillance activities: "Does knowing one's genetic risk make one more or less likely to engage in a program of cancer screening or certain dietary practices?" The focus on surveillance behavior is particularly ironic in the case of breast cancer susceptibility genes because none of the recommended practices, such as mammography or prophylactic mastectomy, are highly effective or appealing. This view of the implications of genetic testing is built on the implicit assumption that the value of good health trumps all other social goods and personal goals.

Very few commentators broaden their attention to include a more general cultural analysis of the background assumptions underlying genetic testing and risk stratification activities. But we argue that the social impact of advances in genetics will ultimately prove more far-reaching and profound than those requiring an immediate policy fix, such as rules preventing employers from conducting tests of prospective workers or legislation preventing discrimination. (Of course, we are not suggesting that enforcing *real* legal protections will be simple or that we oppose the legal reforms that are clearly needed if molecular genetic medicine—whether used for prevention, diagnosis, or treatment—is to have benefits that outweigh potential harms.)

We will next outline some concerns about genomics and risks to which a cultural analysis directs one's attention. The list is not intended to be all-inclusive. We begin by addressing the constructed nature of risk and risk discourse. Our argument derives from the anthropological and sociological literature on risk analysis. The main points are that issues of risk are often narrowly framed and this framing tends to obscure assumptions and values on which risk calculations depend. A number of issues of broad concern tend to be ignored due to the narrow framing of risk concerns. For example, how does genetic risk analysis bear on the cultural construction of group identities and the self?

The Meaning of Risk

There has been considerable research on how lay people understand mathematical risk estimates proffered by scientists. Most of that research has not called into question the fundamental assumptions of risk analysis.

Risk probabilities themselves have been considered accurate; research has focused not on the creation of risk numbers by experts, but on how individuals understand (or misunderstand) the numbers. An alternative perspective is the recognition that risk figures themselves are cultural constructions tied to contexts of professional production. Risk analysis and, more broadly, technology assessment have been commonplace practices for many years, particularly for technologies that are associated with environmental and occupational hazards. The program to examine the ethical, legal, and social implications of genomic technologies involves practices similar to the assessment of environmental risk. Therefore, cultural analysis of existing practices of risk assessment has a bearing on current concerns about genetic risk.[18]

Not surprisingly, those who undertake risk analysis have generally not considered their own cultural assumptions to be relevant to the scientific tasks of risk calculation.[19] A common notion is that one can collect the facts and figures, do the calculations, and derive a measurement of risk that is neutral with respect to cultural assumptions and social interest. However, deriving risk figures is a complex task involving theoretical presuppositions, estimates, incomplete information, and selection.[20] Moreover, there is always a choice to focus on one particular risk rather than some other risk. These choices are inevitably shaped by the cultural and institutional settings in which they are made.[21] In the case of genetic testing for breast cancer, it is impossible to ignore the politicized nature of the response to the breast cancer "epidemic" in the United States when considering the meaning of being at risk. Genetic testing for breast cancer risk has been the topic of intense media scrutiny and aggressive marketing as a medical breakthrough. By contrast, genetic testing for colon cancer risk is much less discussed, in spite of its potentially greater promise in both preventing disease and reducing mortality. The majority of American women seriously overestimate their personal chance of developing breast cancer and assume it strikes at an average age much earlier than is the case; it truly is a dread disease.[22] Interpretation of data about breast cancer risk probabilities, whether by experts or laypersons, takes place against this charged background. We are not suggesting that risk figures are worthless or unscientific, rather, we argue that they are cultural artifacts as well as scientific abstractions. Awareness of this fact is important in understanding the meaning and limitations of risk analysis.

These observations are clearly applicable to current estimates of the genetic risk associated with complex diseases. Despite great advances, the human genome has not yet been "decoded" and, more important, we have barely begun to understand the function of most genes, never mind the complexities of gene-gene and gene-environment interactions. The current genetic risk figures associated with various cancers and other multifactorial diseases are preliminary and will inevitably be revised again and again. For example, the figures cited in the introduction for the risk of breast cancer for women with BRCA1/2 mutations, which are the figures most commonly cited, conflict with other studies based on different populations. In one study the risk of breast cancer associated with BRCA1/2 mutations was found to be 50 percent rather than the often-cited figures of 70 to 85 percent.[23] Bernadine Healy, in an editorial commenting on this study and three others that appeared in the same issue of the *New England Journal of Medicine,* observed that pressures to use these discoveries has led to "bookmaking and fortunetelling" in the absence of factual information about all the variables that affect the development of breast cancer (although Healy appears to have faith that "facts will ultimately preempt statistics").[24]

Even if we were to discount that many people promulgating risk figures have commercial and professional interests, and that the general public often has a ravenous appetite for "medical discoveries," factors that might lead to exaggeration, risk figures should be treated with caution. There are important qualifications that should be appended to all risk figures but which often go unstated. As discussed above, one misleading practice is the application of "risk" numbers derived from populations to provide estimates of risk to individuals in clinical and other settings. The breast cancer figures cited above are sometimes derived from families with a high frequency of breast cancer and in other cases from ethnic groups living in a particular locale. So are these figures applicable to other groups? Possibly not, since we know that the figures derived from different populations vary. And how do you tell who should be counted as belonging to a particular group? Membership in ethnic and "racial" groups is particularly problematic because they are not clear-cut classifications subject to external verification. This matter is often treated in a cursory fashion that ignores the reality that identities are constructed through complex social processes.[25]

Many problems are fundamental to risk assessment, and they are not simply due to a temporary lack of good information, a situation that will be easily corrected as science progresses. Of great importance is the problem alluded to above. There is inherent difficulty in moving from estimates derived from populations to individual risk figures. This problem is generally ignored because it is impossible to surmount. Making guesses based on statistical inference is standard practice. Practitioners understand intellectually and conceptually that each individual is unique and may or may not reflect population-based trends, but in the clinic these risk abstractions take on a life of their own, they are transformed into facts upon which decisions are based. A woman deemed to have a 70 percent risk of breast cancer during her life may experience herself—and may be experienced by her physician—as in danger. This danger is "real" in spite of the likelihood that thirty women out of each one hundred will not develop cancer. Genetic counselors and other clinicians are often frustrated by an individual patient's inability to grasp the complex notions of probability that underlie risk estimates. There is a tendency to view risk in a dichotomous way—either one gets the disease or one does not. Considering the complexity of risk calculation, at one level the resistance of individuals to probabilistic explanations, their tendency to either experience danger or not, makes sense. In this case the lay "resistance" shown to professional understandings of risk accurately reflects the limits of the data.

Given the importance of social and cultural context, how should we approach the issue of lay understandings of risk? A further problem with risk discourse is that it often acts to hide value assumptions in what appear to be objective assessments. Risk estimates are often presented in ways that reduce inherent uncertainties through representational strategies. The very process of taking risk numbers and converting them into colorful graphs and charts presented in easy-to-read patient education brochures creates the idea that the information is *certain*.[26]

Lay understanding may be characterized as irrational when people fail to accept or understand the quantifiable risks, as determined by experts, associated with different activities and decisions (classic examples include public opposition to nuclear power and a host of food production technologies such as bovine growth hormone). However, public "perception" of risk is generally not narrowly tied to numerical calculations, but is framed within a broad social context of potential loses and benefits. Where the physician or public health advocate may be principally concerned with the risk of disease, the individual is likely to evaluate risk estimates within the context of a broad range of other commitments and concerns that relate to values, employment, and relations with family and friends. A young woman concerned about marriage and children, if offered genetic testing for breast cancer risk, may evaluate the numbers very differently than a cancer specialist. The term perception should not be read to indicate that the public simply misperceives expert "knowledge" of risk. Rather, the issue is the interpretive context in which calculations of risk have validity.

The Institutional Imperative of Risk Avoidance

Much of the ethical discussion surrounding the Human Genome Project pays lip service to concerns such as risk (which is not to demean the effort—one could argue that it is an advance over previous efforts to assess the impact of technology). The overwhelming impression is that the implementation of the technology is inevitable and that the only issue is how to make the implementation as painless as possible. That is, there are risks of developing disease (such as breast and ovarian cancer), and these are the primary concern to the political, scientific, and economic institutions involved in the Genome Project. Social consequences that might complicate the investment in information obtained from the Human Genome Project are of secondary importance. From the public's perspective, or more accurately the publics' perspectives, the problem might be different (if there was a choice): "Do we really want and need these technologies?"

One of the important qualities of modern technologies like nuclear power, transportation systems, computer networks, and molecular medicine is that they are deeply embedded in powerful institutions and complex networks of relationships. Technologies such as genetic susceptibility testing do not exist in and of themselves but develop within and take shape from preexisting social structures. There is, therefore, a tendency toward inertia. Medical research centers, public health institutions, biotechnology companies, and governments have particular sets of values and objectives; these are reproduced with each new technologic possibility. This process may in part provide the explanation for the sense that there is little new in the development of molecular medicine and genetic risk analysis, just an extension and deepening of earlier practices. That is, it is easiest to follow the path of least resistance, that which appears from within the local institutional logic as the obvious, the "natural" course of action. In this scenario a test for genetic risk is developed based on scientific breakthroughs, then commercial development is followed by clinical implementation in a natural sequence. From within these institutional frameworks it is very difficult to appreciate the rationality of alternative perspectives or to conceptualize alternatives with a different cultural logic.

One way by which this inertia has tended to operate is through framing risk as a purely quantitative issue. Strictly speaking, risk is a quantitative issue, but in practice, as we have suggested, this is never the case. Moreover, risk quantification is nearly always undertaken to inform public policy, an activity that is ultimately based on judgments of social value, whether recognized or not. From a certain perspective the appearance of neutrality is one of the great attractions of risk analysis: it limits policy debate by reducing discussion to narrow technical issues, ignoring broader social or moral concerns. Although it may be invoked as a conscious strategy, in many cases a quantitative focus is merely the result of a perspective that sees no limits to the extension of scientific rationality. The unexamined cultural logic of the principal institutional actors makes it seem as if once the risk has been established (derived from calculations that are themselves dependent on hidden values) there is an obvious course of action.

Discussions of genetic risk tend to assume that if it is possible to identify persons at heightened risk from a disease and one can effectively intervene to lessen the risks (or in some instances, even if one cannot), then calculating individual risk is necessarily a good thing to do. The assumption is that scientific knowledge and technical control are of primary value. Not all members of society share in these values equally or in every situation. Risks are perceived, understood, ignored, and responded to within social worlds of relationships and beliefs (a fact that is no less true for those with scientific and medical expertise). Merely considering risk from a technical perspective does not do justice to lay understandings and responses to risk.[27] People evaluate and respond to scientific claims according to their values and current circumstances, and by drawing on a wide variety of other sources of information, including information concerning the trustworthiness and reliability of those making risk claims.[28] A genuine understanding of risk needs to be sensitive to these different responses and their own situated logic. However, these responses tend to be hidden in the shadow cast by the dominant risk discourse and where they do see the light of day are often stigmatized as ignorance that must be rectified by better education.

What may be truly risky in genetic susceptibility testing is that lay responses and attitudes toward risk will be disregarded or discounted within a framing established by dominant institutions, including current bioethics practices that promote a simplistic model of decision making. In this model the risks and benefits of a genetic test are meant to be fully disclosed, of course, but little attention is paid to the subtleties of risk discourse, to how much is hidden and how much is deeply uncertain. Decisions by individual patients are too often confined within a narrow technical definition of health. The use of genetic susceptibility tests for population-based health promotion will likely be guided by similar conceptual constraints. The extent to which ethical debate remains narrowly focused on accurate and open disclosure of (seemingly straightforward) risks and benefits illustrates how dependent the debate is on professionals who are themselves caught up in the dominant biomedical paradigm.

The Construction of Group Identity and the Self

The most significant question one can ask about any technology is: What will it do to our sense of ourselves, our sense of others, and our social relationships? Genetic risk analysis hints at many potential changes, some of which we only dimly foresee, and others we may not foresee at all. Before we consider a few of these potential changes, we should rid ourselves of the notion of technology as a mere tool we use to meet various ends, in this case, better health. As Brian Wynne observes, modern forms of technology, "are so all-embracing in their organizational and experiential aspects as to become a way of life itself—we *live* technology rather than use it. [Technologies] come to define the meaning of social interaction."[29] This insight applies not only to the genetic technologies of risk assessment, but also to the statistical apparatus of epidemiology and the media technologies of public health prevention campaigns.

A dilemma that is directly related to risk stratification is the problem of changed cultural meanings of illness due to the chance occurrence of particular disease genes in certain "socially constructed" human subpopulations. Classic examples are sickle cell anemia in Africa and in African Americans and cystic fibrosis in Northern Europeans. These diseases are found in many groups but occur in much higher frequencies in certain subpopulations. Notice that we are purposefully not using the term race, a term anthropologists consider biologically meaningless. A very concrete example of a new disease taking meaning from the population where it occurs is the newly developing association of breast cancer with Ashkenazi Jews of Eastern European origin. If you do a careful reading of the popular press, you will find a growing social construction of breast cancer, particularly the forms of cancer associated with the new genetics, as a "Jewish Disease." This tendency unfortunately pervades the medical literature as well, driven by the early observation that certain mutations in the breast cancer gene—specifically the 185delAG mutation—have been found more frequently in individuals from Jewish backgrounds. No one mentions that the existence of carefully collected blood specimens from Tay Sachs disease screening programs made early identification of this mutation technically feasible. Tay Sachs is a "classic" genetic illness found most commonly in those of Ashkenazi origin (as well as French Canadians and others); repositories of blood from Jewish individuals who had been screened for the Tay Sachs gene made possible the identification of breast cancer gene mutations in this population. Many other relatively isolated human populations also have a high number of idiosyncratic mutations in the breast cancer gene, Finns for example, but this was largely ignored in media accounts. Of course genes are rarely limited to specific populations, rather *frequency* varies among groups.

It may not seem particularly significant that certain diseases become identified with particular human subpopulations, but bear in mind that the consequences of attributing disease risk to particular groups are rarely neutral. The history of genetics (in some eras actual *eugenics*) is replete with examples of the danger of the social use of biological information: the abuses of mandatory sickle cell disease screening programs is the classic story in the United States. Labeling an identifiable subpopulation as "at risk" must always be done with caution. The inverse of this problem is that some individuals who might benefit from genetic testing will be less likely to be offered the test and the follow-up care because their perceived identity means that they do not belong to the "at risk" group.

Another concern is the effect of genetic risk on how one lives with and experiences one's body. As commonly understood, disease risk has many sources. There are environmental risks, such as exposure to lead or other pollutants, that are external to the individual and over which the individual often has little control. Another dimension of risk includes personal characteristics over which one has some control, or partial control. Examples of these "lifestyle" risk factors include diet, exercise, and in the case of breast cancer, age of first pregnancy. Risk identified by genetic diagnostics greatly expands a further category of risk, which has been called "embodied risk."[30] How will women understand risk that literally resides within them, in their genes, over which they have little or no control, and which they may already have passed on to their children? Will breasts and ovaries be experienced as potential time bombs, harboring the early stages of cancer, in need of constant surveillance?

Testing is never simply a matter of gaining knowledge and control over disease. With it comes anxieties, fears, and even, in some cases, ill-health as a consequence of the test.[31] These are particularly acute in the case of embodied risk. Unlike environmental or lifestyle risks, embodied risk resides within one's physical being, is intangible, is not easily accounted for in the usual discourses of risk, and is not amenable to a strategy of control directed by the person at risk.[32] Instead, at-risk individuals are placed in a liminal state betwixt and between health and illness, their body existing as an object of medical surveillance and a constant source of danger.

Widespread attention to genetic risk may greatly extend existing forms of subjectification. No one would be left untouched; the logic of genetic risk is that we are all at risk from at least some of our genes. Pushed to its rational conclusion, everyone would be living in a world of anxiety about genetic risk, including the need for constant surveillance of our bodies for signs of the onset of some dread disease. This despite the fact that most of us would be apparently healthy and have little reason, that is, a reason that would have counted as a reason previously, to be concerned.

One might argue that these problems are simply a consequence of lack of knowledge, that they are an artifact of our inability to act on the knowledge of genetic science in a decisive way, that our current situation is a temporary state, a kind of scientific purgatory.[33] This account suggests that as science advances, each genetic risk will lead to a simple, effective treatment without side effects. Imagine a drug that could prevent the development of breast cancer in all women. (Leave aside for a moment the fact that it might be reasonable to give such a drug to all women, obviating the need for genetic testing.) The reality is likely to be much more complex; we have, of course, no guarantees that particular diseases will be "solved." Drugs powerful enough to prevent the development of cancer will likely have significant "risks" of their own, perhaps leading to the possibility of disease in other organ systems.

Americans in particular already live in a culture of health anxiety and widespread preventive medical testing.[34] Is there no limit to the surveillance we are willing to practice on ourselves and the genetic calculations and predictions we are prepared to do? There is a point where prudence becomes folly. "The body has become a project to be 'worked on' as part of a person's self-identity."[35] Surveillance of this sort may already have come to seem natural enough in our society but for many it has to be an odd behavior for healthy people to engage in. This may change if we continue down the road of genetic susceptibility testing; we may all become selves divided from and permanently unsettled with our physical selves. American society is replete with fears of "big brother," but maybe the most insidious sort of surveillance is the type we willingly accept and practice on ourselves.

Genetic Risk and Personal Responsibility for Health

Another concern surrounds the relationship of public health practices to ideas of individual responsibility. Genetic risk can be seen as an extension of public health concerns that focus on lifestyle risks associated with smoking, diet, sexual behavior, and the like. The difference in this case is that genetic risks would not necessarily be seen as a choice, at least if we are discussing testing of adults for late-onset diseases like cancer and heart disease. However, genetic risks, once identified, might be subject to management through lifestyle choices: regular medical screening, changes in diet, changes in work environment, and so on in order to minimize risk. This is the new paradigm of prevention proposed by the CDC and Dr. Collins. Genetic risk adds to existing public health campaigns by identifying subgroups of the population that are at higher risk of particular diseases and individuals who become targets for education and intervention.

There is an important moral aspect to this culture of self-surveillance, a feature that is apparent in many existing public health campaigns.[36] Susceptibility screening can be seen as part of a broader public health trend in which individuals are exhorted to monitor themselves and take responsibility for their own welfare. It is not merely that one monitors one's health, but that one comes to see one's continued health as one's personal responsibility.[37] Guilt is inevitably a part of this process. If the "experts" have the moral responsibility to provide knowledge; the individual has the responsibility to ensure that he or she is informed and acts on that knowledge. We delude ourselves if we think a coercive dimension can be excluded from these technologies. It may not be coercive in the sense that state-sponsored eugenics programs in the past were coercive, but may act more subtly through our individual sense of self.

Meredith Minkler makes an argument similar to the one we have made with respect to lay responses to risk.[38] She argues that the ideology of personal responsibility for health ignores the social and political context within which individuals live. Contrary to the assumptions implicit in public health campaigns, individual behavior change is difficult to accomplish because, Minkler claims, it oversimplifies complex behaviors. She argues instead for an approach that advocates individual responsibility within a broader social context. Again, what is at issue is whether public health will be sensitive to the varying conditions within which people absorb health issues into their daily lives or whether it will continue the more typical top-down approach that assumes passive absorption of "scientific truth" by a public that is treated as if it exists in a social and cultural vacuum.

The focus on individual risk factors, whether identified as genetic or not, also becomes part of the problematic idea that individuals have full moral responsibility for their own health, that individual action is enough. This model of health promotion and disease prevention deemphasizes the vital importance of the collective practices of governments in protecting the environment, providing safe food and water, or assuring healthy work environments.

Conclusion

Clearly, the burdens created by the need for constant surveillance and risk stratification are real. Efforts to evaluate the ethical, legal, and social implications of the new molecular medicine have not yet adequately addressed these concerns. In the domain of disease prevention and health promotion, the advent of molecular techniques of risk stratification will intensify existing dilemmas. Individuals will be exhorted to take responsibility for their health, to turn their bodies into projects to act on. The health dangers we choose to focus on—inevitably constructed within particular sociocultural and political contexts—will "inevitably include moral judgments of blame."[39] Groups identified as "at risk" may be subject to stigma.

The breast cancer genetics story illustrates another problem: once begun, the practice of risk stratification seems to accelerate in an ever upward spiral. We observed previously that there seems to be no limit to the number of health risks that can be created and that must then be acted upon. However, risk assessment for any particular condition may also generate further efforts at risk stratification rather than a relief of uncertainty. As attempts are made to institute eligibility requirements for BRCA1 and BRCA2 genetic testing, an iterative process is set up whereby the very existence of testing to provide risk information will require ever greater delineation of individual risk. There are strong commercial pressures favoring the use of genetic testing for breast cancer susceptibility in advance of unequivocal evidence of its utility. In part to prevent overuse of genetic testing, critics (including many breast cancer activists) and cautious clinicians recommend that tests be offered only to women at demonstrated high risk due to family history. But how do health plans, or governments, or individual clinicians make decisions about who to test? They develop new models that assign risk numbers to individual women in order to determine eligibility for genetic testing that will give further information about risk.

Anxiety about breast cancer is high. The risk spiral is driven by a deep and widespread cultural fear of breast cancer. A discourse of risk propels women endlessly forward in a quest for more information, while more information often brings with it greater anxiety. Genetic susceptibility testing for breast cancer, with its myriad risk numbers and its arcane calculations, may seem to respond to women's needs for reassurance, information, and certainty. But it does so by ignoring the social burdens of being "at risk," of living a life devoted to disease surveillance. If we fail to examine the implications of genomic science, we blunt our communal awareness of the ways in which we are welcoming the disciplinary practices of biomedicine, and letting our social value and moral worth be judged by our "risk" status and our ability *not* to get sick.

NOTES

1. The first author wishes to thank the Rockefeller Foundation for a residency at the Bellagio Study and Conference Center, where the final draft of this chapter was completed. Both authors wish to thank their colleagues in the Stanford Program in Genomics, Ethics, and Society for many valuable discussions about the promise of molecular medicine.

2. For a review of current knowledge in this area, see Charlie Davison, Sally Mcintyre, and George D. Smith, "The Potential Social Impact of Predictive Genetic Testing for Susceptibility to Common Chronic Diseases: A Review and Proposed Research Agenda," *Sociology of Health & Illness* 16 (1994): 340–71.

3. Shirley Lindenbaum and Margaret Lock, Preface, in *Knowledge, Power and Practice: The Anthropology of Medicine and Everyday Life,* ed. Shirley Lindenbaum and Margaret Lock (Berkeley: University of California Press, 1993).

4. For an earlier discussion see Nancy Press and Barbara Koenig, "Graphing Uncertainty: The Presentation and Representation of Individualized Risk for Breast Cancer" (paper presented at the annual meeting of the American Anthropological Association, San Francisco, Calif., November 1996).

5. For a more comprehensive review, see Barbara A. Koenig et al., "Genetic Testing for BRCA1 and BRCA2: Recommendations of the Stanford Program in Genomics, Ethics, and Society," *Journal of Women's Health* 7 (1998): 531–45.

6. D. F. Easton et al., "Breast Cancer Linkage Consortium. Genetic Linkage Analysis in Familial Breast and Ovarian Cancer: Results from 214 Families," *American Journal of Human Genetics* 52 (1993): 678–701; D. Ford et al., "Genetic Heterogeneity and Penetrance Analysis of the BRCA1 and BRCA2 Genes in Breast Cancer Families," *American Journal of Human Genetics* 62 (1998): 676–89; D. Ford et al., "Breast Cancer Linkage Consortium. Risks of cancer in BRCA1-Mutation Carriers," *Lancet* 343 (1994): 692–95; D. F. Easton, D. Ford, and D. T. Bishop, "Breast and Ovarian Cancer Incidence in BRCA1-Mutation Carriers," *American Journal of Genetics* 56 (1995): 265–71; D. F. Easton et al., "Cancer Risks in Two Large Breast Cancer Families Linked to BRCA2 on Chromosome 13q12–13," *American Journal of Human Genetics* 61 (1997): 120–28.

7. Bettina Schone-Seifert, "Risk," in *Encyclopedia of Bioethics,* rev. ed., ed. Warren T. Reich (New York: Simon & Schuster/Macmillan, 1995), pp. 2316–21.

8. Alan R. Petersen and Deborah Lupton, *The New Public Health: Health and Self in the Age of Risk* (London: Sage, 1996), p. 23.

9. Francis S. Collins, "Preparing Health Professionals for the Genetic Revolution," *JAMA* 278 (1997): 1285–86.

10. Laura M. McConnell et al., "Genetic Testing and Alzheimer Disease: Has the Time Come?" *Nature Medicine* 7 (1998): 757–59.

11. Muin J. Khoury and the Genetics Working Group, "From Genes to Public Health: Applications of Genetics in Disease Prevention," *American Journal of Public Health* 86 (1996): 1717–22.

12. Khoury "From Genes to Public Health," p. 1718.

13. See Richard C. Strohman, "Ancient Genomes, Wise Bodies, Unhealthy People: Limits of a Genetic Paradigm in Biology and Medicine," *Perspectives in Biology and Medicine* 37 (1993): 112–45.

14. Richard Klausner (lecture at the Office of Research on Women's Health, Washington, D.C., 18 November 1997).

15. D. C. Allred et al., "HER-2/neu in Node-negative Breast Cancer: Prognostic Significance of Overexpression by the Presence of in situ Carcinoma," *Journal of Clinical Oncology* 10 (1992): 599–605.

16. B. Dahlback and B. Hildebrand, "Inherited Resistance to Activated Protein C Is Corrected by Anticoagulant Cofactor Activity Found to Be a Property of Factor V," *Proceedings of the National Academy of Sciences* 91 (1994):

1396–1400; J. S. Greengard et al., "Activated Protein C Resistance Caused by Arg506gln Mutation in Factor Va. (Letter)," *Lancet* 343 (1994): 1361–62.

17. Gina Kolata, *Clone: The Road to Dolly, and the Path Ahead* (William Morrow, 1998).

18. The following sections on risk draw on the work of Brian Wynne. See Brian Wynne, "Technology, Risk and Participation: On the Social Treatment of Uncertainty," in *Society, Technology and Risk Assessment,* ed. J. Conrad (London: Academic Press, 1980), pp. 173–208; Brian Wynne, "Risk and Social Learning: Reification and Engagement," in *Social Theories of Risk,* ed. S. Krimsky and D. Golding (New York: Praeger, 1992), pp. 275–97.

19. There are, of course, individuals who have thought deeply about the limitations of techniques of risk assessment. See, for example, William W. Lowrance, *Of Acceptable Risk: Science and the Determination of Safety* (Los Alto, Calif.: William Kaufmann, 1976).

20. Mary Douglas and Aaron Wildavsky, *Risk and Culture: An Essay on the Selection of Technological and Environmental Dangers* (Berkeley: University of California Press, 1982); Mary Douglas, *Risk Acceptability According to the Social Sciences* (New York: Russell Sage Foundation, 1985).

21. See, for example, Diane Vaughan, *The Challenger Launch Decision: Risky Technology, Culture, and Deviance at NASA* (Chicago: University of Chicago Press, 1996).

22. Press and Koenig, "Graphing Uncertainty."

23. J. P. Struewing et al., "The Risk of Cancer Associated with Specific Mutations of BRCA1 and BRCA2 among Ashkenazi Jews," *NEJM* 336 (1997): 1401–08.

24. Bernadine Healy, "BRCA Genes: Bookmaking, Fortunetelling, and Medical Care," *NEJM* 336 (1997): 1448–49.

25. Petersen and Lupton, *The New Public Health,* pp. 37–43.

26. Press and Koenig, "Graphing Uncertainty."

27. See Jon Turney, "The Public Understanding of Genetics: Where Next?" *European Journal of Genetics and Society* 1 (1995): 5–20; Jon Turney, "Public Understanding of Science," *The Lancet* 347 (1996): 1087–90.

28. For a detailed discussion see Lambert and Rose's discussion of people identified at above-average risk of coronary heart disease due to familial hypercholesterolaemia. H. Lambert and H. Rose, "Disembodied Knowledge? Making Sense of Medical Science," in *Misunderstanding Science? The Public Reconstruction of Science and Technology,* ed. Alan Irwin and Brian Wynne (Cambridge: Cambridge University Press, 1996).

29. Wynne, "Technology, Risk and Participation," p. 179.

30. Anne Kavanagh and Dorothy Broom, "Embodied Risk: My Body, Myself?" *Social Science and Medicine* 46 (1998): 437–44.

31. Deborah Lupton, *The Imperative of Health: Public Health and the Regulated Body* (London: Sage, 1995), pp. 92–99.

32. Kavanagh and Broom, "Embodied Risk."

33. Mary-Claire King, the scientist who first identified and named the BRCA1 gene, makes this point. See Koenig, "Genetic Testing for BRCA1 and BRCA2."

34. See Daniel Callahan's arguments about the tyranny of "healthism" in "Freedom, Healthism, and Health Promotion: Finding the Right Balance," in D. Callahan, ed., *Promoting Healthy Behavior: How Much Freedom? Whose Responsibility?* (Washington, D.C.: Georgetown University Press, 2000), pp. 138–152.

35. Petersen and Lupton, *The New Public Health,* p. 23.

36. Deborah Lupton, "Risk as Moral Danger: The Social and Political Functions of Risk Discourse in Public Health," *International Journal of Health Services* 23 (1993): 425–35.

37. Sarah Nettleton, "Governing the Risky Self: How to Become Healthy, Wealthy and Wise," in *Foucault, Health and Medicine,* ed. Alan Petersen and Robin Bunton (London: Routledge, 1997), pp. 207–23.

38. See Meredith Minkler, "Personal Responsibility for Health: Contexts and Controversies," in D. Callahan, ed., *Promoting Healthy Behavior: How Much Freedom? Whose Responsibility?* (Washington, D.C.: Georgetown University Press, 2000), pp. 1–22.

39. Petersen and Lupton, *The New Public Health,* p. 18.

DANIEL CALLAHAN

Freedom, Healthism, and Health Promotion: Finding the Right Balance

To judge by appearances, health promotion and disease prevention are riding high in public and professional esteem. Few would deny their value. Are they not the wave of the future, the key to a healthier population, and a potent way to help control the costs of health care? Have not HMOs embraced health promotion with special enthusiasm, and does not the media offer endless information and advice on how to stay well and be fit? Don't most of our food products now carry nutrition information on labels in great detail, presumably to be devoured by a nervous, conscientious public eager for the latest word on what goes into their stomachs? Is there still a single American alive who does not, at least now and then, feel a pang of guilt (even if no more than that) at some infraction of the multitudinous guidelines to good health with which we are daily bombarded?

There may be less here than meets the eye. For every bit of positive evidence that health promotion and disease prevention are faring well (smoking down) some countervailing evidence can be found pointing in the opposite direction (obesity up). The enthusiasm of health activists to get nutritional information on food labels is surely matched by the indifference of many Americans to reading those labels. For every American serious about living healthy lives, there can probably be found one who could not care less.

What might one conclude from this mixed evidence? At the least it seems reasonable to say that Americans are divided and ambivalent about the health promotion and disease prevention movement. At most it may be possible to say that not only is the public divided, but also that, as a movement, health promotion has still not found the best way to promote itself or to cope well with the diverse range of responses, overt and tacit, that it seems to elicit. I am not sure which is nearer the truth, but I want to explore some major problems with the movement that might offer some fresh ways of thinking about the future of health promotion and disease prevention.

Three problems in particular seem apparent. One that might be termed political is the struggle between those who take a public interest view of health and those who take a libertarian view. A second might be called the medicalization problem—the tension, that is, between a perspective on health that tends to turn unhealthy behavior into a medical problem to be solved by skilled clinical interventions and one that sees most unhealthy behavior as something people bring on themselves and which they can eliminate. The third problem is the scientific one, which pits on one side those who think we already know a great deal about the causes and conditions of good health against those who have grown skeptical or jaded about the validity of any data in the face of a constant flow of contradictory information.

While it would be perfectly possible to treat each of these problems separately my approach will be to fold all of them into what I have here called the political problem. Each of the other problems has, I believe, a distinctive place within, and indeed helps to shape, the political context. I want to present a relatively simple thesis about that political problem, try to show its full dimensions, and then offer some possible ways of dealing with it.

My thesis is this: despite the surface appearance, Americans are fundamentally divided, both politically and within themselves, about health promotion and disease prevention. They are divided in part because there is no clear political consensus on the extent to which government (and other important social institutions) should go to improve health-related behavior; in part because of a strong proclivity in this country to medicalize deviant behaviors that seem to resist education and exhortation; and in part because available scientific information seems bewilderingly able to support just about any position any person cares to take about his or her health. Americans are in general just not certain what role to give the pursuit of health and the avoidance of disease in their lives, and this uncertainty strongly flavors the other ingredients that are part of my tripartite thesis.

The Political Struggle

I want to characterize the political struggle as one pitting two opposed perspectives against each other, one of which I will call the public interest viewpoint, the other the libertarian viewpoint. I don't want to claim that these are entirely tidy categories, or that people decisively adopt one or other of the perspectives. Some of us, including me, are not sure just which perspective best characterizes the way we act. I offer these opposing viewpoints as relatively rough though serviceable categories; what matters is less the purity of identity with one or the other than whether people are inclined—even if not always consistently—one way or the other.

The public interest perspective encompasses three ingredients: an appraisal of personal health as critically important to the good life; a judgment that illness and disease are a major source of social and economic burdens; and a belief that it is a duty of government to do all it can, by social pressure always and legal sanctions when necessary, to promote health and prevent disease.

The war against tobacco of recent decades is the most readily available symbol of the public interest perspective. It is a war waged with an unwillingness to take any prisoners: the use of tobacco is an evil, those who sell and promote it are villains, and the economic and medical costs to society ruinously unacceptable. Those on the front lines of the war are prepared to act as harshly as they can to win the war: there is no sympathy for those who find pleasure in smoking; nothing but scorn for those who would compromise the effort to keep young people from tobacco (in striking contrast to the stance on teenage sexual behavior, where "realism" is espoused, condemnation condemned, and relatively permissive sexual education pursued); and utter contempt for the tobacco manufacturers and purveyors who have hidden or falsified important scientific information, sanctioned addiction, and seduced both the young and the old into deadly habits.

But if the war against tobacco is the most striking manifestation of the public interest perspective, it finds its milder counterparts in many other places. The organized and sophisticated efforts of the government Centers for Disease Control and Prevention (CDC) provide the broadest picture in areas such as HIV/AIDS and injury prevention, the prominent place given to health promotion and disease prevention efforts in federal and state health policy, and the much-touted importance that managed care organizations supposedly give to the subject. But it is a picture that could not sustain itself if it did not build upon a deeply rooted view of human health as an exceedingly high value, one of the highest nonreligious values.

The economic burden of disease—with its emphasis on the costs to the economy of productive life-years lost, or the diminishment brought about by illness and disease—is thought sufficient to justify a strong government intervention. A showing that poor health habits can do harm to others—the effect of driving under the influence of alcohol—provides here too an even more direct rationale for government intervention.

Health promotion, in sum, has behind it the power of a *moral* appeal (helping people avoid the evils of disease), an *economic* appeal (illness and disease are a burden on society), and a *political* appeal (an appropriate role for government, whose task it is to promote the general welfare).

The libertarian perspective moves in a very different direction. While in principle it takes no position on the value of health in human life, in practice it proclaims that there is a higher value: that of personal choice about how to live one's life, including the decision to put it at risk if that is the way one wants to live. Liberty and choice, not health, are the highest human values. To be sure, hang-gliding, fatty foods, a lifestyle heavy on television viewing and low on exercise, are hazardous. So? The point is to be free as one sees fit; that is what gives meaning and dignity to life.

The public interest viewpoint, hanging like a sword of Damocles over our private lives, ready to slice away our most important liberties, is obsessed with health. It wants to make the protection and promotion of health a kind of supreme human good. But how can its proponents possibly proclaim that as a final truth, as if different convictions did not exist? Public interest proponents feel free, in the worst kind of authoritarian way, to impose their version of the good life on the rest of us. No religion would dare, in the face of the doctrine of the separation of church and state, to impose a particular religion upon us as the best way to live our lives. But the forces of what has been termed "healthism" have no such compunction or self-restraining limitations. As pungently defined by the late Czech-British physician Petr Skrabanek

> healthism is a "symptom of political sickness." Extreme versions of health-ism provide a justification for racism, segregation and eugenic control since "healthy" means patriotic, pure, while "unhealthy" equals foreign, polluted. In the weak version of healthism, as encountered in Western democracies the state goes beyond education and information on matters of health and uses propaganda and various forms of coercion to establish norms of a "healthy lifestyle" for all. Human activities are divided into

approved and disapproved, healthy and unhealthy, prescribed and proscribed, responsible and irresponsible.[1]

The purveyors of healthism would have us toe the good health line by
worshiping at the altars of epidemiology, burden-of-illness data, and—
as role models—congenital hypochondriacs who think they can avoid
illness and death if only they avoid the wrong food, the wrong air, and
the wrong romantic companions.

Science, Politics, and Medicalization

The struggle between the public interest and libertarian perspectives
reflects, of course, a larger parallel struggle in American political life.
On the one side are those who believe that government has a perfectly
acceptable role to play in society, and on the other, those who see it
as a menace. Even if in politics more generally the libertarian viewpoint
seems relatively extreme, at the far end of the conservative spectrum,
it has considerable tacit support in the health arena, even among many
who would not call themselves libertarian. That tacit support takes the
form of endless jokes about, and jibes at, the public health perspective.
There are jokes about the lack of scientific consistency, the most common
being those that note a total shift in the evidence, seemingly from week
to week. During the period I was writing this chapter, over a three-
month period there were many revisionary news stories on health risks.
One headline read "Study Shows Obesity Less of a Risk Than Thought."
Another one said "Being Thin While Pregnant Seen As Best," reversing
a couple of decades' advice to the contrary. There are jokes about the
extent to which some state or local governments will go to root out
bad health habits—put those evil smoking teenagers in jail. There are
guffaws about the low risk—far less than the chance of being hit by
lightning—of many alleged dangers, for instance death on California
beaches because of passive smoke and hot cigarette butts in the sand.

An editorial in the British journal *Economist,* commenting on American science and titled "Drop That Steak or We Shoot," observes that
"Death, modern science has discovered, is the leading cause of mortality,
followed closely by folly and freedom. It is thus reassuring to see that
governments are cracking down on all three."[2] And there are few who
can forget the famous Woody Allen film *Sleeper,* where the hero wakes
up from a long sleep to discover that fatty foods have been declared safe.

But that joke has found its real-life counterpart lately in studies
showing that obesity may not be as dangerous as once thought and that

some forms of fatty food may be perfectly healthy to eat and protective against strokes. The problem here is not only that the base of scientific information for health promotion and disease prevention shows itself embarrassingly weak from time to time. It is also that too much health promotion education has seemed to turn all of life into one massive threat, from the food we eat (full of carcinogens, harboring dangerous bacteria) to the air we breathe (rife with nasty particles of something or other). At some point this kind of risk-mongering backfires. Even if the information is accurate—there are risks out there!—a steady diet of it invites regurgitation, either in the form of outright despair or a round of new jokes to take the place of the old ones.

The public interest perspective, not notable for its sense of irony, has simply not learned to cope with this situation. The repeated call for better science and better public education is eminently defensible. But if the "better" science as often as not throws out the earlier worse science—which we were assured last year was true—then the whole venture can look precarious at best and simply hilarious at worst. How, it must be asked, can the health promotion and disease prevention movement learn to deploy scientific information more effectively to avoid those all-too-common pitfalls?

The constant American temptation to medicalize persistent social problems does not help either. Whatever the exact truth about the role of obesity in causing or exacerbating poor health, it is certainly true that obesity has been turned into one more medical problem. People don't just eat too much, or exercise too little; many, it is said, may be genetically predisposed to obesity, or suffering from a pathologically slow metabolism, or whatever. Thus a principal message of the health promotion movement—that people can take charge of themselves and live healthy lives—is at least partially undercut. The antismoking campaign can have a similar subversive effect: If tobacco is addictive (and made deliberately more addictive by cunning tobacco companies), then it is simply cruel to expect people to kick the habit; they need technical assistance in the form of counseling, patches, and the like.

A curious, even seductive logic seems to come into play when educational efforts to change behavior fail: there must be some deeper force at work, amenable only to a medical approach and effectively dispossessing people of their self-determination. Even among those who have no reason to believe they are somehow medical victims, either of genetics or addiction, it is easy to succumb to the idea that even they perhaps are dealing with something larger than themselves, as if their life and their health are not entirely in their own hands. But is our life and health in our own hands?

Is to Know the Good to Do the Good?

It was Socrates who contended that "to know the good is to do the good," and philosophers have ever since been arguing about the truth of that claim. If we *really* know what's good for us, will we do it? Or, if the truth about our own good is too painful, will we do whatever we want, persuading ourselves against counterevidence that it is *really* good for us?

All this is pertinent to health promotion. If most people by now have at least a rudimentary knowledge of what will advance and what will harm their health, and if most cannot claim to be victims of uncontrollable forces and desires, then why is it so hard to do that which they know they should do? Two possible reasons are worth consideration, one focusing on the external circumstances of people's lives, the second on the frequently self-made difficulty of doing that which we would have ourselves do, as when we convince ourselves that harmful behavior is good, or at least worth a gamble.

External Circumstances

A conference I attended in the city of Naples, Italy, in the summer of 1996 made vivid for me the power of external circumstances in shaping people's behavior. On the positive side of the ledger was the fact that few people on the streets were obese, despite the readily available delights of southern Italian cooking. But even so, why should they be obese? Most walked to where they were going rather than taking cars. The typical city buildings were multidwellings some five and six stories, all without elevators; no need for stairmaster machines in those apartments. Even the food, though heavy on pastas, was not fatty; and wine was drunk—and everyone drank some—in moderation. On the negative side, the pollution from autos, buses, and motor scooters was palpable; a thick haze hung in the air. Motor scooters were more common than cars, but not one driver in 1,000 wore a helmet (actually I saw none at all). Whole families, babies, husbands and wives—also without helmets—drove at high speed through the streets, indifferent to lines painted down the middle of those streets.

I was seeing a way of life, some of it conducive to good health, built into the daily life of people, and some of it unhealthy, no less built into their daily round. An improvement in the health status of the citizens of Naples would have required a resistance to those modern devices known as autos and elevators, control by law of the emissions of those autos in use, and a radical job of education, backed by legal sanctions, on the value of helmets for those riding motor scooters. My casual impression in talking to the Italians was that they would be happy to have more cars and elevators, that they would possibly accept some control of emissions, but that they would not under few, if any, circumstances welcome helmets. They were not curious about, much less obsessed with, head injury data. They liked the freedom of riding with nothing on their heads; and if that was dangerous, so be it. You have to die from something. No evidence of any strenuous effort to control tobacco was in evidence either, though the Italian government recognizes the problem.

I have no doubt that comparable descriptions could be developed of other ways of life. Health-related behavior will be a function of a way of life, more or less amenable, or more or less resistant, to conscious efforts to change that life to improve health. Cultural values or simply long-ingrained practices will explain the variations from one place to another. In the United States we are permissive about fast food restaurants, harshly puritanical about smoking, in love with the auto despite its obvious deprecations, and erratic in our effort to control air and water pollution. What the field of health promotion and disease prevention lacks is a systematic way of looking at these cultural and social patterns and figuring out how best to intervene in them. What I have labeled "external circumstances" seem in some cases to be a deep part of a people's way of life, and in other cases simply the result of historical circumstances that could be changed with little public resistance.

The Difficulty of Doing That Which We Would Do

Many of the external circumstances I have just noted would make it difficult for people who are part of that world and way of life to go against the behavioral grain. I say "difficult," not impossible. People can and do give up smoking in Naples, even though there is comparatively little social pressure to do so; many work to control their drinking habits, and with success. Even in the United States there are people who manage to walk, not drive, to get to the other side of the street. We can change the way we live, even if that sometimes requires fighting the tide of social pressure, or custom, or simply psychological inertia. Sometimes victims should not be blamed—when there are profound obstacles standing in their way of a kind few people manage to transcend. But sometimes victims should be blamed when it is evident that other people similarly situated do manage to change their behavior. If they can do it, why can't others?

But why do we sometimes persist in doing that which we know is likely to hurt us and which we wish we were not doing? No doubt one possible answer is simply that it is hard to change, to give up a way of life, or a habit, that seems a basic part of us. We manage, I suspect, to persuade ourselves—or at least one part of the self persuades another part of the self—that the harmful behavior is somehow indispensable to our self-identity (e.g., the sense of added social security that smoking seems to give some people); we persuade ourselves, that is, that the bad is the good, or that not all that seems bad is truly bad.

Another possible reason for risky behavior is that we persuade ourselves that the gamble is worth taking, a statistical risk of harm in order to gain an immediate pleasure. There is no utter certainty that a diet too rich in fat will kill us; it simply shifts the long-term odds in a hazardous direction. But we know that passing up a fine meal of old-fashioned French cuisine will immediately deprive us of pleasure.

It is at this point the many jokes about health promotion and disease prevention have their bite: we are being asked to live a certain kind of tiresomely austere life, abiding by some specific, often difficult, rules of good health. In return, we are promised (well, not quite *promised* it turns out when we read the fine print) that we will have long and healthy lives. But the risks are usually statistical with the worst outcomes often low in probability, the science weakly based or downright faulty, and the demands for self-discipline high, even daunting. We can also be fairly sure, at least once a year, of hearing a media story about someone alive at 103 who attributes her long life (and it is usually "her" not "his" life) to drinking, smoking, and enjoying life. And during that same year one of our nonsmoking friends will die of lung cancer.

It takes a very dedicated person to exercise regularly, to always eat properly balanced meals, and to avoid all occasions of potential harm. To be sure, it is possible to find a kind of *via media* here: now and then failing to exercise, now and then eating the wrong food, now and then pursuing hazardous sports. But that *via media* itself can require considerable discipline: not letting the periodic deviations become more common and from there becoming a habit. Unfortunately, I speak here more from personal experience than I would like, and I have noticed that I am not alone.

Health and Happiness

To begin musing on some of the ironies and paradoxes of the pursuit of good health, as I have been doing here, eventually drives one back to a basic and difficult question, or rather two related questions. What is the relationship between health and a happy life? To what extent should those parts of life that bring some pleasure and happiness be sacrificed in the name of promoting good health?

Commonplace observation of our neighbors shows that there is no perfect correlation between health and happiness. Many healthy people are unhappy for reasons having nothing to do with their health (thwarted ambition, failed marriage, lack of purpose in life, etc.). And many unhealthy people are happy, for reasons that allow them to transcend and endure their ill health (sometimes because they have rather stoic temperaments, sometimes because their other gifts do not require good health or an able body—I think here of the scientist Stephen Hawkins). Beyond some point of course poor health can utterly obviate the possibility of happiness or any sense of well-being. But it is both interesting and mysterious that this line is drawn at different places for different people; disease alone does not appear utterly decisive (though chronic depression and chronic pain come about as close to that as possible).

Now if there is some truth in my generalizations about the troubling lack of perfect symmetry between health and happiness, then it is not irrational to come to a practical conclusion about living our lives: it makes no sense to pursue good health and avoid risk obsessively. Such a quest cannot guarantee that the health we gain will make us happier (or even result in a good health outcome), nor does it guarantee that we will of necessity come to some unhappy end if we fail to assiduously pursue good health. The (wise) truth of the matter is that there may be many things in life more worthy of pursuit than perfect health, and some of them may be risky.

The downhill skier greatly enhances the danger of injury or death compared with simply taking a nice thirty-minute walk each day (assuming a proper arm swing for maximum benefit, of course). But the skier gains great pleasure, gets vigorous exercise, and has a diverting hobby that can be followed for many years. That's not a bad trade-off or necessarily a reckless way to live. At the least, exercise seems a matter best left to individual choice. The same can be said for choosing not to exercise and to watch one's weight; not everyone will, nor is there a moral law that everyone should want to trade off other pleasures and values for the sake of promoting health.

Let it be understood here that I am not espousing the regular taking of risks or the neglect of health. I am simply trying to understand why so many people can feel ambivalent, and even hostile, to a health promotion and disease prevention movement that presumes to have a definitive answer to the question of what is good to do, or not to do, in the name of health. It often has neither definitive answers scientifically about the route to good health nor moral answers about the appropriate level of zeal in pursuing that route; and even if it has the former in some cases, they do not necessarily entail the latter in all cases.

If the health promotion movement fails to take that uncertainty into account, it invites ambivalence at the least and hostile rejection at the worst. Its message should be: *if* you want to maintain good health (and there are some good reasons to want that), then here are some *likely* (not certain) ways of doing so; and *if* you want to ignore some *reasonable* guidelines for maintaining good health, be sure you are prepared to accept the resulting harm to yourself, and perhaps to others as well, if you incur injury or illness.

Some Proposed Guidelines

I want to try now to suggest some guidelines for the health promotion and disease prevention movement, designed to respond to the problems I have raised in this chapter. They are meant to address this question: Is there a way of resolving, or ameliorating, the tension between the public interest and the libertarian perspectives? If not, the movement will remain in serious trouble, failing to achieve its potential. I have contended that both of these perspectives have deep roots in our society as a whole and are expressed in the lives of individuals trying to decide what place to give the pursuit of health.

Stance and Tone

The stance of the health promotion movement should be one of confidence that there is much that can be done to improve the health of individuals and of the population as a whole. It should, however, be modest and circumspect—even as it is persistent—in pressing its case. It should neither imply greater credibility for its scientific claims than can reasonably be sustained nor hector and intimidate people to change their unhealthy behavior. Particularly objectionable are draconian legal measures, such as recent laws in some states that create criminal penalties against teenage smoking. This approach, even if effective in reducing smoking, could well create a future generation of libertarians, hostile to zealous health promotion. The banning of smoking in all public places based on the supposed danger of passive smoke (which lacks full scientific support) may also turn out to be a short-sighted view.

Health promotion efforts should take the long-term view, asking not only what might work to improve health-related behavior in specific instances, but also what approaches will best preserve the credibility and good civic name of health promotion and disease prevention activities. The danger of a backlash—whether out of anger or simple fatigue—should never be underestimated. It may well explain some of the current difficulties of health promotion efforts in making real progress.

Good Health as Freedom Enhancing

It should never be assumed that waving the flag of good health will instantly excite people. Many people who engage in less than healthy behavior usually believe that they have a good reason for doing so. They are rarely unaware of the risks inherent in their behavior but they have convinced themselves that there are respectable reasons—given their values and life goals—for doing so. Hence, it seems imperative that educational programs find ways to stress two points. One is that efforts to improve one's health will enhance rather than restrict one's freedom and sense of well-being. People who give up smoking often feel immediately better as well as immediately relieved of the strain of feeding an addiction; and that can be as telling a reality as the less-palpable reduction of long-term harm (which they might not have experienced anyway).

The second point is that people rationalize their bad health behavior. It is the reasons people give themselves for the behavior that have to be dealt with head-on, all the ways we fool ourselves into thinking that what we want to do is what is good for us (or at least not as dangerous as assorted authorities say) or worth the risk. Careful research to identify those rationalizations, and then clever ways of countering them, seems imperative.

Benefits to the Community

The environmental movement has demonstrated that it is possible to persuade people to act in the name of the common good, and it has no less helped to show them that such action is imperative on occasion. Successful health promotion and disease prevention programs can make a significant contribution to population health. The American public can understand that well enough when there is the possibility of an outbreak of food poisoning, polluted water, and dangerous viruses. Much more needs to be done to help them see that their personal health behavior can, in concert with the behavior of others, have a powerful impact on the health of the community, for good or ill.

This will not be an easy educational campaign, for the obvious reason that the contribution of any given individual will not make a great statistical difference. There is none of the immediacy or drama of an individual who is the carrier of a dangerous infection. But here the success of the environmental movement in changing individual behavior when no one person's behavior makes that much difference is an instructive example. The impact of individual health behavior on their families, on overall health care costs, and on health care facilities can be made palpable. Best of all, a solid case can be made that here at least is a kind of invisible hand at work: individuals acting in their own health interest will, when others do the same, make a direct contribution to the health of the entire community.

Sustainable Medicine

Contemporary high-technology medicine, aiming at curing or ameliorating the condition of those already sick, or screening them to detect a risk of disease, is turning out to be an unsustainable enterprise everywhere in the world. The combination of aging populations burdened by chronic and degenerative disease and an expensive high-technology response is laying an increasingly heavy burden on health care systems—systems that now seem to be approaching a chronic crisis and an endless series of reforms attempting to deal with that crisis. The thrust of twentieth-century scientific medicine, which has sought endless and open-ended medical progress and technological innovation, is becoming economically insupportable, producing marginal health gains at ever higher costs.

Something else will have to take its place: a sustainable medicine, by which I mean a medicine that sooner rather than later finds a steady-state plateau at an affordable level and, at the same time, can provide real promise of decent health for most people through the life cycle.[3] Health promotion and disease prevention—together with a corresponding shift from an individual-centered to a population health-centered approach—offer the only viable prospect of generating a sustainable medicine. A population-centered approach will require a greatly increased effort at improving the socioeconomic conditions conducive to good population health.

It will no less require a stronger focus on individual responsibility for health—which is not in the end, nor can it be, incompatible with a focus on population health factors. The concern now that too heavy an individual focus both blames the victim and naively overlooks the social determinants of health can only be met by taking those determinants more seriously. Yet in the end a test of the success of taking that route will be that individuals both can and do act in ways conducive to good health. Not all affluent, educated people have good health habits, even when they know better; nor do all poor people have poor health habits, even when they have been poorly educated about their health.

No country can in the long run depend on simply throwing technology at illness and disease. The movement toward evidence-based medicine and the recognition of the need to ration the costly use of technology are necessary first steps to a sustainable medicine. The necessary next steps are to find a way to bring population-based medicine to the fore and, with it, a more sophisticated set of health promotion and disease prevention strategies.

Health and Anti-Health

I have tried to show that the struggle between a public interest and a libertarian perspective on health promotion is deep and serious. It touches not simply on different ways people think about health in their lives but also the way they think about personal responsibility and choice and about the role of government in their lives. Health promotion has not been typically thought of as one of the battlefields of the American culture wars. It would be wise, however, to recognize that it is, even if the external manifestations of that war seem less dramatic and visible than they are in many other areas—and of course in a few areas, such as teenage pregnancy, health promotion is already well caught up in those wars.

The problem is how to minimize the cultural struggle and, perhaps more urgently, to do everything possible to help it steer clear of the nastier, more egregious struggles that now mark the cultural wars in other areas. While I think it fair to say that the war is already on with health promotion, it is at an early stage—a stage at which, to use the jargon of the field, considerable primary prevention to avoid an all-out conflict and some secondary prevention to circumscribe the struggles already underway, are still possible.

While it may seem trite to say, the health promotion and disease prevention movement most of all needs to find a middle way. If a neglect of personal health and an indifference to the social determinants of health are serious dangers, healthism also carries its own striking dangers, not the least of which is its capacity to generate a nasty, mocking (but often covert) backlash at a movement that can all too easily invite such a response. If the way to good personal health is prudence, balance, and common sense, not organized hypochondria; the way to a successful health promotion movement is likely to lie in exactly the same direction.

I have tried to think of a motto, and here are two possibilities. "Work hard to stay healthy, which is possible, but don't be inordinately fearful of getting sick, which is inevitable." Alternatively, "No life is survivable without some respect for risks to health, and no life is worth living without occasionally running some of those risks."

NOTES

1. Petr Skabanek, *The Death of Humane Medicine and the Rise of Coercive Healthism* (London: Social Affairs Unit, 1994), p. 15.

2. "Drop That Steak or We Shoot," *Economist* (December 13, 1997), p. 15.

3. This is the general theme of my book *False Hopes: Why America's Quest for Perfect Health Is a Recipe for Failure* (New York: Simon and Schuster, 1998).

Daniel Callahan, Barbara Koenig,
and Meredith Minkler

Promoting Health and Preventing Disease: Ethical Demands and Social Challenges

Could it be said that health promotion and disease prevention are the health care strategies of the future—and always will be?[1] There is good reason to ask that wry, ironic question. On the surface, these strategies seem to have come into their own, encouraging hopes that they will shortly become the chosen pathway to societal health.

Is it not the case that the media is full of information and advice on how to stay healthy and avoid disease?

Is it not true also that the managed care revolution, now providing a growing proportion of all health care, has given a prominent place to health promotion and disease prevention (which we will simply call health promotion for the remainder of this chapter)?

And is it not evident when the scientific data are consulted that the combination of public health programs and behavioral change account for much, if not most, of the greatly improved health status of Americans over the past century?[2]

If all of this is accurate, why is there any reason to doubt the eventual dominance of health promotion strategies in health care policy? How can one doubt that they are the wave of the future? All too easily.

In the United States, national expenditures on public health comprise less than 5 percent of total annual health care spending.[3] There is considerable doubt as well about the strength and persistence of the managed care interest in health promotion; they could well become the first victims of harsh competitive pressures among HMOs. As the former president of the American Public Health Association has pointed out, when helping enrollees adapt health-promoting behaviors requires "substantial investment," and when the average enrollee switches plans every few years, the cost-conscious HMO may well ask itself why it should invest in smoking cessation or exercise programs when some other plan will reap the benefits down the line.[4]

For all of its interest in health promotion, the media may well confuse people as much as enlighten them, as one story contradicts another, one piece of advice counters another piece of advice, and what's in and what's out in the name of health can sometimes seem to change faster than the weather.

But the most discouraging phenomenon is simply this: despite decades of efforts to improve health-related behavior, the evidence of success is decidedly mixed—and getting worse of late in many areas. Smoking in general is down, but teenage smoking is showing a disturbing increase once again. Among eighth, tenth, and twelfth graders, the proportion of youths who smoke daily increased by almost 50 percent between 1991 and 1996, with 20 percent of twelfth graders now smoking on a daily basis.[5] The exercise surge of the 1970s and 1980s, once thought a new and secure part of our common life, also appears to be on the decline. Fewer, not more, people do any regular exercise, with over 60 percent of adults refraining from any regular physical exercise and fully one-quarter leading sedentary lives.[6] Despite recent declines, our teenage pregnancy rate remains the highest in the advanced industrial worlds, with close to a half million teens giving birth annually.[7] Or consider what has been called the French paradox: "The French, eating foods deemed by Americans to be fattening and fatal, are thinner and live longer than Americans, while we, growing ever more obsessed with 'healthy' low-fat foods, are as a nation growing fatter—the American paradox."[8]

No panaceas for these distressing trends are in sight. In that respect, the future of health promotion is by no means assured. Or better, there is no assurance that it will gain the dominance and prominence its supporters have always projected for it. It could remain the eternal success of the future, a future that somehow never quite arrives or is always over the next hill. An impasse has been reached.

The contention of this chapter—the outcome of a two-year study conducted by The Hastings Center and the Stanford University Center for Bioethics—is that a fresh recognition of three factors is necessary for health promotion to move beyond the present impasse.

The first factor is a new awareness of the cultural and political context of health promotion efforts, most notably the enormous tension between a common good, public health perspective and the individualism, even libertarianism, that continued to dominate the mainstream of American culture in the late twentieth century.[9] At the same time, if health promotion is to gain political and public support, it must find ways to make more credible its contribution to the economics of health care and to the actual health of the public.

The second need is for a clear-eyed assessment of the power, ever-growing, of a narrow medical perspective on disease and illness that stresses biological reductionism (with molecular genetics the research vehicle of choice), technological innovation, and individual health, ordinarily through rescue medicine. This perspective is directly aided and abetted by the rising power of for-profit medicine and health care.

The third requirement is a careful examination of the various ethical options open to government, employers, and managed care organizations to change unhealthy behavior patterns. Moral exhortation and public "education" are still the tactics of choice for much of the traditional health promotion movement. Something more potent is needed.

We do not mean to suggest that the three needs we have identified are the only ones of importance. Instead, we argue that if promotion and disease prevention are to take their rightful and forceful place in health care, then far greater attention must be paid to the social, cultural, political, and moral dimensions of efforts to improve the health of the public. A focus on technique alone is not doing, nor can it do, the necessary work.

Freedom, Healthism, and Health Promotion

The drive for improved public health has always faced cultural obstacles. Public health programs lack the glamour of high-technology medical interventions, and the focus on population health as opposed to individual health contradicts basic tenets of American individualism. These trends have become more acute in recent decades, as technology and freedom are celebrated. A critical tension lies at the heart of this problem: the plausibility of the public health case over the difficulty of making it effective.[10] There appears, for instance, to be a wide and strong public awareness that the way a person lives his or her life can have both a direct and indirect impact on health. Driving while intoxicated can lead directly to death, while a paucity of exercise can bring about the same result more slowly and insidiously, usually in combination with other poor health habits. There is no public outcry against that message.

But it is not always a congenial or easy message to live by. It can require a self-discipline and self-denial that are not easy if needed over a period of years, if not decades. For another, the work, family, and leisure habits and the socioeconomic and environmental burdens of contemporary life work against that self-discipline. As Jonathan Robinson has pointed out, when our culture continues to say to us "Why walk when you can ride?", when it urges us to get every new labor-saving device and to not leave our chair even to change a television channel or our computer to send a fax, is it any wonder that the notion of building in thirty minutes of exercise three or four times a week goes against the grain?[11] Life is hard enough, and rushed enough, and demanding enough already without having to keep a tight rein on the hungry, tired, lazy, and buffeted self. Our social and occupational ways of life often work against good health habits, even if there is a strong will to pursue them. The decline in exercise of late provides some striking testimony to the difficulties here.[12]

There is also some evidence of backlash underway, partly because of the difficulty of living in a healthy way, and partly perhaps as a kind of ideological protest. The late Czech-born English physician Petr Skrabanek spoke as forcefully as anyone about the dangers of "health-ism." "The pursuit of health," he wrote, "is a symptom of unhealth." And "when this pursuit is no longer a personal yearning but part of state ideology, *healthism* for short, it becomes a symptom of political sickness. . . . Human activities are divided into approved and disapproved, healthy and unhealthy, prescribed and proscribed, responsible and irresponsible."[13]

If the libertarianism espoused by Skrabanek—keep the nanny state out of our health affairs—has few explicit supporters, it surely has many tacit adherents. Their presence is felt in the many, almost epidemic, number of jokes made about the obsessive pursuit of health—the years of good life lost to the boredom of jogging, for instance; or the remark of one wit who said "When I am tempted to exercise I lie down until it passes"; or the endless bantering about the irresistibility—"You can't live forever"—of one more serving of rich, tasty food. It consists also of that other category of jokes, too close to the truth to be dismissed out of hand, about the unreliability of "expert" health advice, given one year and rescinded the next. Just what is too much salt anyway? And how can one fail to groan or laugh just a little over the recent discovery that fat in the diet may actually help prevent stroke rather than cause it?

A tacit libertarianism—reacting to an overemphasis on health as "the paramount virtue of society"[14]—may also be reflected in the large number of people who are voting with their stomachs when they decide to eat what they like come what may, or with their legs when they vote to turn on the television instead of taking a walk. While the "pro-choice" Smokers Alliance may be the best organized of the groups trying to keep the government away from health-related behavior, there are legions of the nonorganized who simply ignore what the government, a notorious spoilsport, has to say about the way we live our lives.

In pointing out how widespread and powerful is the combination of a libertarian ideology and the difficulty of living a healthy life, our aim is simply to underscore the formidable barriers that now exist on the road to good community health. If it would be a mistake to ignore them, it would be no less a mistake to think they will easily be overcome. The alternative point of view, which we espouse, and which might be called the public interest perspective, is far easier to make than to implement.

What is that perspective? It might best be characterized by noting three of its prominent features. The first is that it takes a population viewpoint on health: it is the health of the community as a whole that is at stake, not just the health of an individual. It notes the large burden of illness and disability brought about by poor health, social conditions, and lifestyle habits, and the cost of that burden to the community as a whole. Moreover, as the transmission of tuberculosis shows, our own health is often contingent on the health of those around us.

Its second feature, however, is to note that individuals as well as the community benefit from a healthy way of life: pain, suffering, disability, and a premature death can thereby be reduced. Individuals will feel better and function better if they live well, and they will do less harm to others.

Its third feature is that it offers a clear alternative to the medical and sickness model of health care that still remains dominant in health care. That model pursues technological innovation, usually expensive, as the best weapon against disease and disability and embraces rescue medicine as the characteristic response to illness. It focuses excessively on individual health and well-being, thereby ignoring the fact that the good health of a community reflects far more than the availability of technological medicine. At the same time, the medical model characteristically offers those individuals marginal gains only—longer lives in poor health—rather than the more radical transformation made possible by successful disease prevention.

Can a public interest perspective be made plausible and politically potent? We believe so, but the first steps require two insights. The first is that the backlash against healthism be taken with full seriousness. A person who lives only for health, consumed with anguish and fear about the possibility of getting sick, is a legitimate figure of fun, and good sport has been had for centuries with hypochondriacs and what Arthur Barsky recently has called the "worried well."[15] The phenomenon of "doing better and feeling worse," noted by Dr. John Knowles two decades ago, is worth more than a raised eyebrow of concern.[16] Hardly less important is an awareness of the rapidity with which the American people can respond with furious negativity when they feel the government has gone too far in trying to tell them how to live. The rapid organization of opposition in California against a new law banning smoking in bars provides just one recent example.

The second insight is the necessity to set health promotion in the context of a philosophy of science (especially the role of epidemiology) and government (particularly the relationship of individual and common good). What is the relationship of health promotion to the common good?

The Good of Health and
The Common Good

Although its history radically antedates the rise of Western individualism, the Hippocratic tradition in medicine has behind it a philosophy of the primacy of individual patient welfare, even though that tradition also took seriously environmental influences on health. The focus of medicine is the good health of the individual patient, a good that transcends all other considerations. This philosophy helped put in place the centrality of the doctor-patient relationship. Individual patient welfare has been a noble and important tradition.

The tradition of public health by contrast, of much later origin, looks upon health as a collective good, changing the angle of vision from that of the individual to that of the community. That tradition is meant to complement the Hippocratic perspective, emphasizing the need for social and political action to promote health and prevent disease in the community as well as recognize the socioeconomic determinants of health.

The moral foundation of the public health tradition is that of human solidarity in the face of the threats of illness and death, and one of its prime aspirations is that of equity of access to a healthy social environment. Together these moral roots and aspirations give a place of honor to the common good, its animating principle. Health promotion can be understood as a common effort of people to fit a vision of good health into a larger vision of a good society.[17]

This way of looking at public health—expressed most eloquently in the World Health Organization's Ottawa Charter for Health Promotion—emphasizes the need for governmental action, for a good and mutually respectful relationship between health professionals and community groups, and for policies that are pragmatic, active, and engaged. In the language of the Ottawa Charter, health promotion indeed represents "a mediating strategy between people and their environments, synthesizing personal choice and social responsibility in health."[18] By virtue of the key perception that disease and poor health have social no less than biological determinants, the public health perspective requires the mobilization of a wide range of community and government resources. The interdependence of people in sickness and in health requires their political and social interdependence in promoting good health.

But Can It Work?

In recent years health promotion as a movement has gained increased professional support and public enthusiasm. HMOs, for instance, often feature their health promotion efforts as part of their competitive effort and marketing techniques to gain subscribers. Not all that support and enthusiasm is based, however, on an affection for those values sketched above that we believe lie at the roots of its most compelling claim on our interest. Instead, a more concrete set of claims has been advanced: that health promotion will reduce health care costs and produce a better cost-benefit ratio than more main-line forms of medical care. Not only are those claims widely believed, they are also thought to be politically most effective.

Despite the political expediency of such claims, some skepticism is in order, and for two reasons. One of them is simply that of truth: if they are false or exaggerated claims they ought not to be advanced as a tactic to gain public support, however advantageous that might seem. The second is that in a society that is already jaded about fluctuating, scientifically insecure health claims, there is a serious danger of cynicism if public doubts begin to rise about the validity of health-promotion claims. For both of these reasons, it is critical that the arguments and evidence and claims advanced in behalf of health promotion be well founded and carefully nuanced. The short-term risk of that approach may be to dampen some of the enthusiasm for health promotion, but the long-term benefit in securing solid credibility is a more important consideration.

What is the truth? We believe three propositions are defensible. The first is that there is little if any evidence that health promotion programs will, of their nature, save money. When the CDC examined some 2,000 health promotion interventions, only a handful—such as influenza vaccines for the elderly and early prenatal care for low-income teens—resulted in actual cost savings.[19] Contrary to the rhetoric that prevention equals savings, the costs of massive education programs to improve specific forms of bad health behavior can far exceed the costs of providing medical treatment for those who succumb to that behavior. Screening and other preventive programs can cost prohibitive amounts of money for each life saved. Given such economic realities, it is hazardously misleading and sometimes downright false to look to health promotion in general as a way of lowering costs.[20] This is an argument that should be permanently retired from public and political use.

The second proposition is that a more solid case can be made for the cost-effectiveness of health-promotion strategies compared with other ways money might be spent to improve health. Cost-effectiveness and cost-reduction are often confused or conflated. Health promotion programs, as an instance of the former, can represent a sensible way of expending resources, and in many cases better ways than alternative possibilities of spending money to improve health. They may also, quite apart from direct financial contributions, help to reduce suffering. Care and caution are needed here. Strategies that are thought to be, or hoped to be, cost effective should always be forced to run a gauntlet of critical and probing questions; cost-effectiveness should never be taken for granted.

The third proposition is that the key to a good overall health care policy is that of finding the right mix of public health strategies on the one hand, and traditional medical strategies on the other. It is tempting for health-promotion enthusiasts to set up a tension between their approach and that of the main-line medicine. That is a mistake. Even with the best imaginable health-promotion policies and programs, people will continue to get sick, to be injured, to physically decline with age, and to die. All that such programs can hope to do is to reduce the incidence of illness, lower rates of premature death, and hold off disability. But that means there will always remain a strong and central role for medicine. We need health promotion to help us to stay well, which is possible; and we need medicine to help us when we are sick, which is inevitable. Economically speaking, a good mix of public health and medicine will help to manage costs in the most efficacious way.

Promoting Health, Changing Behavior

If there are some important uncertainties and ambiguities about the economic implications of health promotion, that is no less the case with its ethical implications. As noted earlier, there is at least one group of people who believe in principle that it is wrong for the government (and presumably for employers as well) to attempt to change people's behavior or to pass any judgment on the way people manage their health. Fortunately, this belief is not the dominant view. But there is no doubt that efforts to change the way people live—and what they do with their bodies—can raise serious ethical issues.

The most obvious and ancient of such issues is finding the right balance between a need to protect civil liberties and the need to protect the health of the public. When does the protection of the public's health justify restrictions on individual liberty? Until recently, a standard response to public health threats, particularly plagues and communicable diseases, was to put the good of the community ahead of the liberties of individuals. Sometimes that bias had good effects—as with the evacuation of Philadelphia in the late eighteenth century during yellow fever epidemics and nineteenth-century efforts in London to control cholera. In other cases, however, prejudice and poor scientific knowledge produced considerable harm in the name of public health, such as the assault on Jews in medieval Europe to control Black Death and the quarantine of Chinatown in San Francisco in the early 1900s to control bubonic plague.[21] Even so, it was until recently taken for granted that the health of the public almost automatically justified the suppression of civil liberties.

The late twentieth century has seen an important shift toward a greater sensitivity to civil liberties. It was undoubtedly the AIDS crisis, emerging in public awareness in the mid-1980s, that helped bring about that shift. As a result of the political pressure brought by those at risk of further stigmatization and social harm as a result of being labeled HIV positive, AIDS was almost from the start treated as a civil liberties emergency with public health implications rather than as a public health emergency with consequences for civil liberties.[22] The AIDS scenario represents the first time in the United States that contact tracing, mandatory testing, and other standard public health measures for treating a lethal infectious disease were ignored.

More recently it has been recognized that what has been called "AIDS exceptionalism" has been too little concerned with the effects of a civil liberties dominance on the health of others, as seen in efforts to adopt a more interventionist approach with women at risk for bearing HIV-infected babies. The latter stance argues that women's civil liberties should not be protected at the expense of their babies, whose lives could be saved and their health improved by an early course of AZT treatment. The troubling outcomes of an overriding emphasis on individual freedom versus public health have also been witnessed in recent struggles within the gay community about the persistence of (and in some communities, the increase in) unsafe sexual practices.[23] Yet even with such trends, older attitudes persist: the CDC AIDS hotline encourages HIV-positive individuals to "think about" telling their partners that they are infected rather than emphasizing their moral obligation to do so in the interest of protecting others from contracting and dying of the disease. A resurgence of tuberculosis has also brought forth calls for a stronger public health stance, even at the cost of some civil liberties of those so afflicted.

There can be circumstances under which a rigorous and strong public health stance is justifiable: when there is a severe and immediate threat to the health of the public; when every effort to avoid a draconian approach has been carefully evaluated and, if possible, tried; and when the restriction of civil liberties is the minimal amount necessary to achieve the desired public protection. The burden of proof should be on those who want to override civil liberties, but it should not be a burden impossibly difficult to meet. In some imaginable cases, there may be little time to develop a nuanced emergency response. Action may have to be taken, and quickly. The possibility of new infectious diseases or plagues in the future is not a matter of science fiction. It is possible and, even worse, likely, as the hazard of the ebola virus should have reminded us.

Personal Responsibility for Health

If there can be occasions when civil liberties may legitimately be restricted in the name of public health, what are we to make of the way people manage their own health? Are individuals to be held responsible for their health-related behavior?

This question is not easy to answer. It touches in a complex way on two important western convictions, not easily reconcilable. On the one hand, we in the west believe that people should be free to live their own lives and to make their own choices about crucial aspects of their existence (and we believe it with particular intensity in the United States); and we no less believe that people have the capacity to make free choices. The basic premise of most health promotion programs is that this basic freedom *can* be exercised in favor of healthy rather than unhealthy ways of life. It is possible to exercise health-promoting rather than disease-inviting behavior. It has been estimated that some 50 percent of illness and death in the United States can be traced to health-related behavior;[24] good health is not wholly or primarily a matter of accident and genetic good luck. It is our doing as well.

Yet individual choice and behavior do not exist in a social vacuum. Income, education, race, and social class correlate directly with health status, and often in ways not causally evident. As the Whitehall study has shown, an affluent person of high social status who also happens to be a heavy smoker is less likely to contract lung cancer than a poor person who smokes. Residence in neighborhoods plagued with persistent poverty has been shown to dramatically increase mortality rates, even when such traditional risk factors as smoking, diet, and exercise have been controlled for.[25] We also know that socioeconomic status is transformed by racism.[26] African-Americans with the same work experience and education as whites have lower incomes, higher costs for goods and services, and more exposure to occupational hazards and carcinogens than whites.[27] Of course people are influenced by their friends, their family, the media, and the cultural context of which they are a part. If this applies to the way they dress, the kind of car they drive, and the food they eat, it also applies to their smoking, drinking, and eating habits.

For all these reasons, sophisticated health promotion programs take as a first premise that the social context of people's lives must be changed if there is to be any serious chance of changing their individual behavior. People can and do stop smoking on their own, but it is easier for them if their family members and friends don't smoke, if they can't smoke in their workplace, and if the taxes on cigarettes makes buying tobacco products exceedingly expensive.

It is not easy to find the right balance between these two perceptions, the one bearing on the capacity for freedom and choice in the face of outside pressures, and the other bearing on the probabilities that people in large numbers will rise above their social environment. One camp has been prepared over the years to self-consciously blame the victim, to tolerate health stigmatization, and to assume that, with will and determination, people can do that which is good for them, which is not all that hard to grasp anyway. The other camp, fearful of that kind of oppressive healthism and its insensitivity to social pressures on free choice, has been prone to think that nothing but radical social change can make any real difference. And there is, conveniently enough, some evidence to support each camp, just enough to keep them going.[28]

There is an alternative to those polarized viewpoints. It is possible both to affirm the possibility of choice while also recognizing the power of context and environment to compromise its actual expression. This alternative can be achieved by programs of health promotion that simultaneously (a) work to have individuals take responsibility for their health-related behavior and (b) work no less hard to change the social conditions that work against such responsibility. An example of such an ecological approach can be found in the violence prevention program in Boston. Developed by physician Deborah Prothow-Stith and her colleagues,[29] the program teaches youth in high-risk neighborhoods new ways of coping with their anger and aggressive feelings and helps them explore the root causes of violence in poverty, racism, and in a culture where the most popular heroes have "Rambo hearts and Terminator heads."[30] But the program also works to mobilize government, business, and the mass media, developing broad-based, multilevel attacks on the problem of violence. These efforts appear to be paying off. Working on both the individual and the broader systems level, and breaking down traditional turf lines between police, the courts, schools, churches, and nonprofit health and youth agencies, the "Boston model" of crime prevention has received much credit for the city's recent and unprecedented twenty-nine months without a single murder among its children or adolescents.[31]

The test of a serious program will be the extent to which it takes up this dual responsibility. In any specific health campaign, to be sure, it will often be far harder to change environments and contexts than to mount educational programs directed at individual behavior modification. That point may well be acknowledged without thereby washing one's hands of the obligation to do whatever can feasibly be done about that situation—which is the long-term, most important requirement.

Economic and Other Incentives for Behavior Change

If there is a range of steps that might be taken to change harmful social contexts, there is no less a range of possibilities in trying to influence individual behavior. They run along a continuum from coercion through manipulation, seduction, and persuasive education to a "neutral" just-the-facts approach. Fear can be employed, incentives and disincentives can be devised, self-interest or altruism can be invoked.

In light of all these possibilities, a basic question can be asked: Who has the right to do what to whom in the name of better health? With the exception of earlier quarantines, where coercion was directly and unhesitatingly used, only in the case of smoking have we seen of late the use of unabashed social, economic, and legal pressure. Smokers are increasingly quarantined by being forced to take their smoking outside or to special areas, economically pressured by high taxes on their tobacco or forced to pay higher insurance premiums, and socially stigmatized by their strong-willed colleagues, neighbors, and even strangers. State laws that bring fines or even jail for underage smokers are explicitly punitive. These methods verge, we might surmise, on the kind of coercive healthism that could well bring a backlash, but have not so far done so in any serious way.

But because ill health caused by tobacco is so clear-cut compared with other behavior, smoking is an exception to general practice. More common are milder forms of incentives and disincentives, many of them deployed by employers, insurers, or HMOs. For the most part, they do not raise serious moral difficulties, except at two extremes. One extreme, discussed with some frequency (even if not all that much practiced), is that of an outright denial of health care to those who are believed to have brought harm upon themselves: smokers, substance abusers, the sexually careless, or those who engage in dangerous recreational activities, such as skydiving.

While this desire for a punitive response may be understandable, it should not be acted upon. One of the oldest and most honored principles of medical ethics is that physicians should minister to the sick regardless of the causes of that sickness. Hence, there has been a long-standing duty to treat wounded enemies in wartime, criminals and other miscreants in peacetime, and all sick people at all times. Behind this tradition lies a perception that it can be exceedingly difficult to determine causality and culpability for illness or injury and that, in any case, it is wrong to combine the role of moral judge and medical healer. The doctor-patient relationship requires that the doctor be trusted by the patient, something that would rapidly become unlikely if doctors began discriminating between worthy and unworthy patients.

No such tradition exists in the case of insurers or employers, though by extension some of the same considerations will apply: a refusal to let physicians treat, or be reimbursed for treating, those who have engaged in unhealthy behavior compromises the integrity of the physician. Neither insurers nor employers, for that matter, are in any position to make definitive judgments on the culpability of sick people for their sickness. No more than the rest of us do they have knowledge of who is free and who is not. For them to enter the business of post hoc judgments would as likely tarnish their reputations as save them money.

We are not saying that insurers or providers have no legitimate means at their disposal to influence behavior.[32] Financial incentives in the form of reduced fees or insurance costs, or disincentives in the form of higher premiums and greater out-of-pocket expenses for those whose behavior puts them at risk, can be acceptable enough. Such incentives must, however, be clearly specified in contractual agreement, equitably applied, and stop well short of being punitively coercive. Forcing people into a bad bargain is no more acceptable in health care policies than in any other realm of human relationships. Nor should the argument that such disincentives disproportionately affect the poor be dismissed either.

Risk and Predictive Medicine

Health promotion and disease prevention have, as public health strategies, always depended heavily upon a calculation of probabilities. A person who smokes heavily over a long period of time has an increased probability of lung cancer or heart disease, just as an obese person has an increased probability of contracting diabetes. But there has been a long-standing problem with that method of calculating risk: it tells us too little about the risk to a given individual. Many heavy smokers do not get lung cancer or heart disease and many obese people do not contract diabetes. The public seems also to have caught on to that anomaly, often preferring the risky Russian roulette of unhealthy behavior to the austerities of clean living. Many win the gamble, beating the odds; and some people who don't smoke get lung cancer, which just goes to show that the course of a life is not a predictable event.

That may be about to change. The growing sophistication of individualized risk analysis—the precision of molecular diagnosis made possible by the Human Genome Project—offers the prospect of pinpointing with greater certainty the risk probabilities for individuals in a way never before possible.[33] This analysis is happening with breast cancer and Alzheimer's disease, two notable examples, and will happen with other common diseases in the future. Yet it offers, for the most part, only a more precise set of probabilities, never utter certainty; and in some cases, moreover, as with early-onset Alzheimer's, predictive genetic testing can offer nothing more than advance knowledge of a coming medical condition for which little can be done.

There is considerable disagreement about whether information alone should be counted as a benefit, and considerable variation in response among (prospective) patients about whether they want, or should have, knowledge of such probabilities. Further, the social and psychological cost of a lifetime lived with the knowledge of increased disease risk remains largely unexamined. In the quest for precise risk estimates, the potential burden of public health practices based on a discourse of risk has not been examined. Predictive medicine, moreover, is already raising serious issues about confidentiality and the uses of such knowledge by such interested parties as insurers and employers.

Still unknown at this time is the likely effect that this increase in individualized predictive medicine will have on efforts to alter the general social determinants of ill health. Possibly it could make the problem seem to be exclusively that of the individual, not also of the society, which would be a harmful turn to predictive medicine. Will the idea that each person has a unique, individual risk profile undermine the sense of social solidarity needed to support the health of the public? It is no less possible that the cost of new molecular preventive techniques could add significant costs to health care, skewing their benefits toward the affluent, reinforcing the current maldistribution of health care resources.

Final Thoughts

The purpose of this chapter was not to resolve many ethical and social issues touched upon in the preceding chapters. It is more imperative at the moment to signal the existence of a number of problems that have not been sufficiently explored and may have critical implications for policy. Because health promotion seems so utterly commonsensical and immediately persuasive, it has been all to easy to see the problems standing in its way as technical matters only: how to devise and implement effective programs and policies.

But it should be clear by now that efforts to improve health, to change personal habits, and to work on unhealthy environmental and social determinants of injury and disease touch on some fundamental questions of morality and politics: the role of government, the place of health in individual and community life, the use of force or persuasion to change behavior, and the vision of society that lies behind a concern for health in the first place. These dimensions of the problem of promoting good health have not gone unremarked, but they have not been explored with the seriousness and depth that they deserve.

The fact that so many efforts to improve health behavior have failed, that progress in health promotion is so difficult, and that there may now be something of a public backlash against what many perceive to be an officious healthism signals the need to bring those dimensions to the foreground. If the idea of "ways of life, ways of health" is true, then what is needed is nothing less than a more comprehensive analysis of the interplay of societal values and health values.

NOTES

1. This chapter is the result of a joint project carried out by The Hastings Center and the Stanford University Center for Biomedical Ethics. It was supported by a grant from the California Wellness Foundation and the Walter and Elise Haas Fund. We would also like to thank the following project participants for their contribution to our project: Ron Labonte, Haavi Morreim, Beverly Ovrebo, Ann Robertson, and Helen Schauffler.

2. Institute of Medicine, *The Future of Public Health* (Washington, D.C.: National Academy Press, 1998).

3. M. J. McGinnis and W. H. Foege, "Actual Causes of Death in the United States," *JAMA* 270 (1993): 2207–12.

4. E. R. Brown, "With Managed Care, What Role for Public Health?" *Nation's Health* (April 1996).

5. T. E. Novotny, "Smoking among Black and White Youth: Differences that Matter," *Annals of Epidemiology* 6 (1996): 474–75.

6. Centers for Disease Control and Prevention, The President's Council on Physical Fitness and Sports, *Physical Activity and Health: A Report of The*

Surgeon General (Washington, D.C.: U.S. Department of Health and Human Services, 1994).

7. S. Ventura, S. C. Curtin, and T. J. Mathews, *Teenage Births in the United States: National and State Trends, 1990–1996* (Washington, D.C.: National Center for Health Statistics, Report PHS 98-1120, April 1998).

8. D. Johnson, "American Pie," *The New York Review of Books,* 18 December 1997, 20–23, at 20.

9. Ronald Labonte, "Health Promotion and the Common Good," in D. Callahan, ed., *Promoting Healthy Behavior: How Much Freedom? Whose Responsibility?* (Washington, D.C.: Georgetown University Press, 2000), pp. 95–115; D. Callahan, *False Hopes: Why America's Quest for Perfect Health Is a Recipe for Failure* (New York: Simon and Schuster, 1998).

10. D. Callahan, *False Hopes.*

11. J. Robison, "Changing Health Behaviors: We Know What to Do to Be Healthy: Why Don't We Do It?" (paper presented at the Art and Sciences of Health Promotion Conference, Orlando, Fla., 8 October 1995).

12. Centers for Disease Control and Prevention, The President's Council on Physical Fitness and Sports, *Physical Activity and Health.*

13. P. Skrabanek, *The Death of Humane Medicine and the Rise of Coercive Healthism* (London: Social Affairs Unit, 1994), p. 15.

14. M. Becker, "The Tyranny of Health Promotion," *Public Health Reviews* 14 (1986): 15–23.

15. A. J. Barsky, *Worried Sick: Our Troubled Quest for Wellness* (Boston: Little, Brown, 1988).

16. J. Knowles, "The Responsibility of the Individual," in *Doing Better and Feeling Worse: Health in the United States,* ed. J. Knowles (New York: W. W. Norton, 1977).

17. A. Robertson, "Health Promotion and the Common Good: Reflections on the Politics of Need," in D. Callahan, ed., *Promoting Healthy Behavior: How Much Freedom? Whose Responsibility?* (Washington, D.C.: Georgetown University Press, 2000), pp. 76–94.

18. World Health Organization, *Ottawa Charter for Health Promotion* (Copenhagen: Author, 1986).

19. U.S. Department of Health and Human Services, *An Ounce of Prevention: What Are the Returns?* (Atlanta, Ga.: Centers for Disease Control and Prevention, 1993).

20. H. H. Schauffler, "The Credibility of Claims for the Economic Benefits of Health Promotion," in D. Callahan, ed., *Promoting Healthy Behavior: How Much Freedom? Whose Responsibility?* (Washington, D.C.: Georgetown University Press, 2000), pp. 37–55.

21. A. Kraut, *Silent Travelers: Genes, Germs and the Immigrant Menace* (New York: Basic Books, 1994).

22. B. Ovrebo, "Health Promotion and Civil Liberties: The Price of Freedoms and the Price of Health," in D. Callahan, ed., *Promoting Healthy*

Behavior: How Much Freedom? Whose Responsibility? (Washington, D.C.: Georgetown University Press, 2000), pp. 23–36.

23. L. Gostin and Z. Lazzarini, *Human Rights and Health and Public Health in the AIDS Pandemic* (New York: Oxford University Press, 1997); D. Wohlfeiler, "Community Organizing and Community Building among Gay and Bisexual Men: The Stop AIDS Project," in *Community Organizing and Community Building for Health,* ed. M. Minkler (New Brunswick, N.J.: Rutgers University Press, 1997).

24. Institute of Medicine, *The Future of Public Health;* M. J. McGinnis and W. H. Foege, "Actual Causes of Death in the United States."

25. M. Haan, G. Kaplan, and T. Camacho, "Poverty and Health: Prospective Evidence from the Alameda County Study," *American Journal of Epidemiology* 125 (1987): 989–98.

26. D. R. Williams, R. Lavisso-Mourey, and R. C. Warren, "The Concept of Race and Health Status in America," *Public Health Reports* 109 (1994): 29.

27. M. Haan, G. Kaplan, and T. Camacho, "Poverty and Health"; D. R. Williams, R. Lavisso-Mourey, and R. C. Warren, "The Concept of Race and Health Status in America," 25, 29; J. Robison, "Racial Inequality and the Probability of Occupation-Related Injury or Illness," *Milbank Quarterly* 62 (1984): 567–90.

28. M. Minkler, "Personal Responsibility for Health: Context and Controversies," in D. Callahan, ed., *Promoting Healthy Behavior: How Much Freedom? Whose Responsibility?* (Washington, D.C.: Georgetown University Press, 2000), pp. 1–22.

29. D. Prowthow-Stith, "The Epidemic of Youth Violence in America: Using Public Health Prevention Strategies to Prevent Violence," *Journal of Health Care for the Poor and Underserved* 6, no. 2 (1995): 95.

30. D. Prowthow-Stith, "Violence Prevention with Youth" (keynote presentation for the Annual Conference of the American Journal of Health Promotion, Orlando, Fla., 20 March 1995).

31. C. Tucker, "Boston Shows How to Deal with Teens," *San Francisco Chronicle* 20 (December 1997), sec. A, p. 20.

32. E. H. Morreim, "Sticks and Carrots and Baseball Bats: Economic and other Incentives to Modify Health Behavior," in D. Callahan, ed., *Promoting Healthy Behavior: How Much Freedom? Whose Responsibility?* (Washington, D.C.: Georgetown University Press, 2000), pp. 56–75.

33. B. Koenig and A. Stockdale, "The Promise of Molecular Medicine in Preventing Disease: Examining the Burden of Genetic Risk," in D. Callahan, ed., *Promoting Healthy Behavior: How Much Freedom? Whose Responsibility?* (Washington, D.C.: Georgetown University Press, 2000), pp. 116–137.

Contributors

DANIEL CALLAHAN is director of international programs at The Hastings Center in Garrison, New York.

BARBARA KOENIG is executive director of the Stanford University Center for Biomedical Ethics in Palo Alto, California.

RONALD LABONTE is president of Commonitas Consulting in Kingston, Ontario, Canada.

MEREDITH MINKLER is professor and chair of health and social behavior at the School of Public Health, University of California, Berkeley.

E. HAAVI MORREIM is a professor in the department of human values and ethics at the University of Tennessee College of Medicine in Memphis, Tennessee.

BEVERLY OVREBO is a professor in the department of health education at San Francisco State University in San Francisco, California.

ANN ROBERTSON is a professor in the department of behavioral medicine at the University of Toronto, Ontario, Canada.

HELEN HALPIN SCHAUFFLER is an associate professor in the School of Public Health at the University of California, Berkeley.

ALAN STOCKDALE is a senior research and development associate at the Center of Applied Ethics and Professional Practice at the Education Development Center in Newton, Massachusetts.

Index